The Venus Dilemma

by Robert Helmer, M.D.

Nash Publishing, Los Angeles

Library of Congress Catalog Card Number: 73-83533
International Standard Book Number: 0-8402-1328-X

Published simultaneously in the United States and Canada
by Nash Publishing Corporation, 9255 Sunset Boulevard
Los Angeles, California 90069

Printed in the United States of America

First Printing

To my co-author and editor, Brett Howard, my appreciation for study and research.

PREFACE

The author's customary habit of dedicating a book to an individual or to a group of individuals is being bypassed in *The Venus Dilemma.* It can, in truth, only be dedicated to Venus herself "trapped by her prey."

It was Catullus who first observed: "Not unknown am I to the Goddess Venus who mingles with her cares a sweet bitterness."

Since *The Venus Dilemma* is a documentary study of venereal disease, it is appropriate that the book be dedicated to the world of lovers, young and old, black and white and yellow and red, male and female, heterosexual and homosexual, in order that they may become acquainted with some of the dilemmas associated with the love sicknesses of the world.

In an antibiotic medical era, many misconceptions regarding venereal diseases—from contagion to cure—exist. Because of the wonder drug, penicillin, the two most common venereal diseases, syphilis and gonorrhea, have been ignored for an entire generation. The apparently sudden outburst that has reached epidemic proportions in certain geographical and sociological areas of our society makes it almost mandatory that *The Venus Dilemma* be a book dedicated to lovers—wherever they are.

It has been said "let love be without dissimulation." It is in such a spirit that *The Venus Dilemma* has been written—not to frighten or distort sexual love, but to inform and enlighten all human beings regarding the past, present, and future role of venereal diseases in our daily lives and in our intercommunal existence.

Robert Helmer, M.D.

CONTENTS

the Venus Dilemma

MARGARET'S CONTRIBUTION
TO GONORRHEA:
THE GENEALOGY OF AN EPIDEMIC

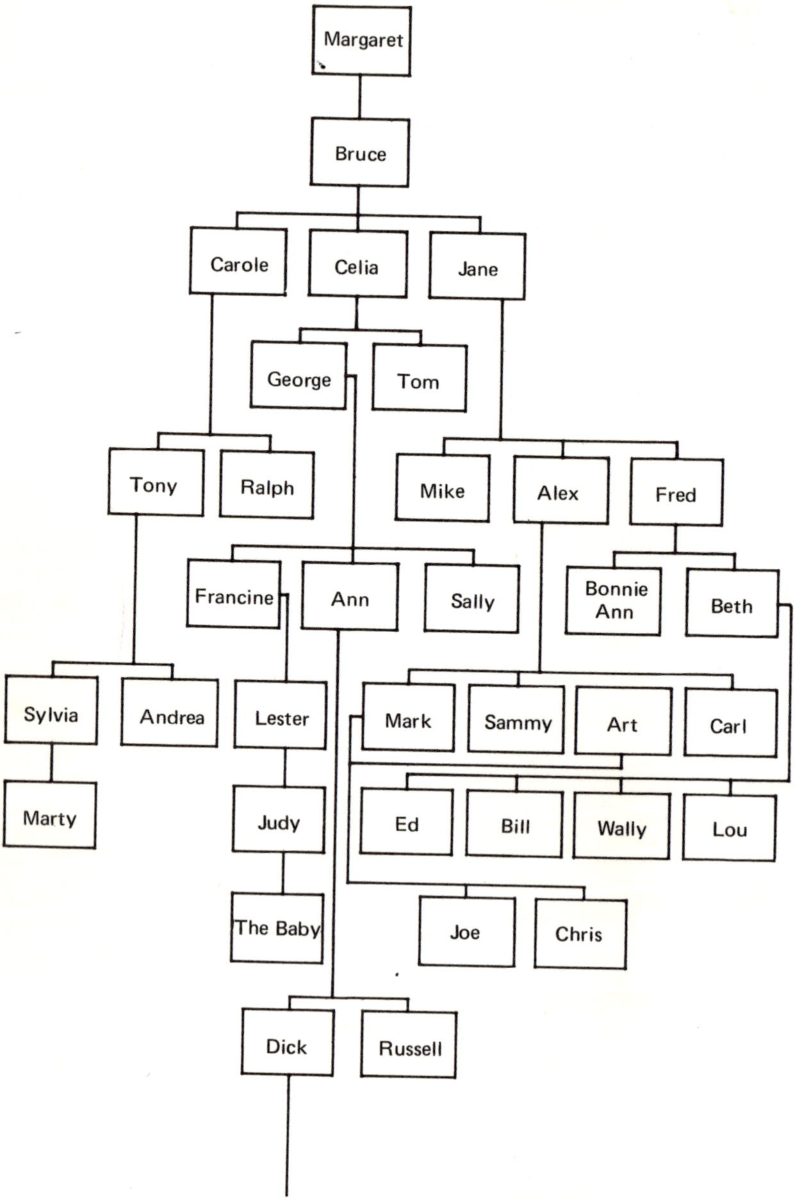

1

WHY VD?

That VD is currently on the rampage again is a fact recognized by physicians the world over. Although some progress in its control had been made in past years, the present-day outlook is bleak indeed.

VD—venereal disease—has plagued man through the centuries: *Gonorrhea* has been recorded by historians since biblical days; *syphilis* is generally recognized as a more recent phenomenon that swept through Europe in the epidemic of the "great pox" at the end of the fifteenth century.

The incidence, morbidity, and mortality that are results of venereal disease, make it imperative that the story of VD become as "social" in areas of communication as the "social" diseases themselves. It is time that each individual become acquainted with the story of VD and all of its sundry ramifications. Each person has a right to know the gigantic efforts of mankind which have been thrust into attempts to solve the problem of VD. Each person has a right to be aware of the tragedies, the frustrations, the impacts of VD upon the lives of human beings, individually and in groups.

VD is *the* human disease; the common scourge of all men of all times.

It is time to determine why man has failed to control and eradicate VD. It is by knowing the entire story, with its confusions and complications, both medical and sociological, that we can be prepared to battle the enemy at every turn.

Let us begin at the beginning. The word *venereal* stems from the name of Venus, the love goddess. Human beings are the only animals that "love all the year around"–and are prone to sexual debauchery. And human beings are the only animals that contract diseases which, because of their usual methods of transfer, are called–*venereal diseases.*

In medical terms, the adjective "venereal" broadly includes any disease transmitted by means of the genital organs. The words "by means of" make the category large enough to include many diseases that are not necessarily transmitted by sexual contact, and, since they do not exist under the stigma of the two most commonplace–syphilis and gonorrhea–it hardly seems proper to list them together. However, the category VD is important and sustained by medical authorities because most diseases included in the grouping can rarely be transmitted through any other means than sexual contact. In most instances, the determination of the true identity of a genital infection can only be ascertained by a qualified physician observing the responsible culprit under a microscope.

Disease is probably as old as human life itself, and as ancient as the life it affects. The parasites that impede us today are, in all probability, sycophants that evolved with man, and some of the diseases of man must have been present thousands of years before the historical record began.

The question of the origin of VD has two aspects: *When* and *how?*

When is history.

How is biology.

Both are incorporated into the story of medicine, man, and VD, both are ancient and contemporary.

Gonorrhea, the more common and the more prevalent of the two most prominent venereal diseases, is caused by the gonococcus, a member of the common class of parasitic bacteria that have cohabited with man since time immemorial. The gonococcus, magnified a little more than a thousand times, looks like a partly deflated balloon, a little smaller than the head of a pin, punched in on one side. Usually, the gonococci are found in pairs, with the punched-in sides adhered together. As we shall see, the evidence of the disease parallels the history of man.

Syphilis is less common than gonorrhea, but definitely more serious. The microbe of syphilis is a moving, bending, wriggling screwshaped varmint called a spirochete. Under the same magnification used for the gonococcus, it appears to be about a half-inch long but is so thin that even when magnified a thousand times or more it is nearly invisible except with the use of special microscopic methods.

The organism of syphilis, the spirochete *Treponema pallidum,* is a Spirillum requiring moisture and tissue for survival. It is able to grow and live despite body defense, but dies quickly when removed from tissue and moisture. Because of its inability to survive on inanimate objects, we can, to a large extent, discount as not authenticated most of the reported cases of transmission by indirect means such as doorknobs, toilet seats, dishes, etc. The essential physiologic secretions (vaginal, salivary, and seminal fluid) collected in all stages of the disease, both early and late, have been shown in controlled experiments to be noninfectious. The blood and lymph tissues, however, may contain the organism in abundance in the early years of infection and at irregular intervals in the later years. From these sources, the organism may be discharged into the fetal circulation during the early stages of pregnancy or into the vaginal tract by way of the menstrual blood. The organism does not survive in the vaginal tract after menses are completed unless lesions are present from which the organism is repeatedly discharged.

Reduced to its simplest terms, transmission of syphilis is a lesion-to-lesion affair except by means of the blood. Unfortunately, the transmitting lesion is often painless, inconspicuous, or hidden. Infectious syphilis generally denotes the primary and secondary stages.

Interestingly enough, the microorganisms of venereal disease are very weak and incredibly fastidious! They grow only in man, and outside his tissues they do not grow but are killed almost instantaneously. Mere soap and water are highly efficient venereal germicides. As a paraphrase of the old song goes: "The love bug will get you if you don't wash out!"

The microbes' inability to survive outside the tissues of man make it highly improbable that they are obtained except by intimate contact. Consequently a drinking glass or a toilet seat are not very convincing as reservoirs of infection. It is almost impossible, for example, to grow the organisms of syphilis in an artificial environment. It is in this context that all diseases known as venereal, however much they differ, are linked together by the social, cultural, and emotional oddities of human sexual behavior.

It is unfortunately true that women have always unjustly borne the brunt of being the purveyors of VD, largely through prostitution. Regardless of how the infection started we must recognize that sexual promiscuity, not prostitution per se, is the major source of the propagation of VD. Unfortunately, the sexually promiscuous person comes in contact with the innocent and passes on the disease, making it imperative in the control of VD that the source of infection be identified. Although woman is traditionally regarded as the purveyor of VD, she is also the child-producing member of society, and for the sake of her unborn children she should be enlightened early in life as to its contagion and its consequences. For many obvious and practical reasons, the sexual education of the female is more important than the sexual education of the male, yet our social mores kept VD a subject taboo for women who were not professional prostitutes, whereas their husbands were supposedly alerted. In reality, the ignorance of the male sex, combined with the imposed ignorance of their wives and the mothers of their children, created one of the social and marital dilemmas of society.

That we have advanced remarkably in the control of infectious diseases cannot be denied, especially when we realize that effective control of infectious diseases did not begin until the nineteenth century. Yet, it is obvious to any student of history that VD was by-passed at that time. Why?

Modern disease control belongs to Louis Pasteur and Robert Koch, who demonstrated that specific types of germs that breed true are, without doubt, responsible for certain specific diseases. Finally, the cause had become *real!*

Previously, the presumed causes of disease had been abstract, supernatural, or fantastic. The germ theory of Pasteur and Koch abolished any existing doubts about contagion. Disease could be transferred from person to person. And in many diseases, this is exactly how they were exchanged. For example, the discovery of Pasteur and Koch confirmed the suspicion of the older Oliver Wendell Holmes, physician and author, that childbed fever (a big killer in its day) was carried on the hands of the doctors who neglected to wash before delivering a woman of her child. Ignaz Semmelweiss, in Vienna, demonstrated that childbed fever could be prevented—if doctors would wash their hands. But both men were derided until Pasteur went before the French Academy and with a crayon drew a string of beads—a chain of streptococci—the cause of childbed fever. The germ theory substantiated William Budd's theory that typhoid fever was carried by human feces into drinking water, or on the hands into food to be consumed. Yet, it was well into the nineteenth century before contagion was no longer disputed. It took the microscope and experiments with microbes and animals finally to resolve the dispute.

In the beginning, the idea of contagion was almost always

associated with Divine Wrath—identified with the miraculous, the mysterious, the supernatural. Epidemics were outbursts of anger on behalf of a godhead determined to punish man.

The very nature of VD and its entanglements with sex is one of the most important elements of the story and is the answer as to why VD was bypassed in the basic history of contagion. The unwillingness or inability of men to deal with diseases relevant to the most driving force in man—his sexuality—has made the problem of coping with VD more difficult than the problems associated with other contagious diseases.

That human sexual intercourse should produce disease, and that disease should be regarded as just punishment for an act of nature odious to the gods or godheads, is a belief completely in accord with man's primitive religious beliefs and the early development of monogamy. In promiscuity, man discovered disease and consequent sterility, and he set about to establish a set of morals for himself, peculiar to himself; that it is not a sin to respond to the urge for sex—the urge for man to reproduce himself is normal—but it is a sin to gratify that desire in such a manner as to jeopardize the well-being of the offspring.

This theory has existed since the very early recorded history of man and is still propounded: that venereal disease is peculiar to man and is contracted through sexual encounters which affect the reproductive organs; and that it must be the issue of the wrath of God, evoked by man's immoral behavior! No other theory was rational or acceptable. Even the scientific facts of the contagious transmission of disease could not penetrate the hard-core facets of Victorian morality. Not even Sigmund Freud, advancing with his emancipating theories of man and man's sexuality, created too effective a breach in the wall of prejudice against separating venereal disease from sin.

In the story of VD, we must interlock a major medical problem with the mystique of man's sexual behavior which is as old and as baffling as the entire history of man. Centuries of inbred religious, racial, and social taboos are involved in what is essentially a medical subject, but which, to date, has not been allowed to be treated as such.

In 1929 an event occurred which should have altered the VD picture and brought it into a positive focus. Ironically, almost a half century later, the dilemma of venereal disease is more pressing than it was during that significant moment in history when Sir Alexander Fleming and Sir Howard Florey were responsible for one of those scientific "accidents" that led to a resoundingly great discovery—the inactivation of infectious organisms by the use of an antibiotic.

Penicillium notatum was a low fungus that grew upon bread which was stale, rotten citrus fruits and melons, certain types of cheeses, and even upon the human skin. Since the beginning of the study of bacteriology, men of science cursed it vehemently when they observed the *Penicillium notatum* taking over assiduously tended laboratory cultures, luxuriating in profusion over the organisms meant to grow there.

Yet, no one had ever asked "Why?" until, one day, Fleming seized upon the idea: "If the green fungus will immobolize these disease microbes, I wonder if it will restrain the same germs when they attack man?"

He proceeded to find out by making a crude extract of a fungus and injecting it into the abdominal cavity of mice that had been inoculated with lethal microbes. They all lived, but the control mice that had been given no penicillin died! Never before had a substance obtained from a living, growing microorganism been used to combat other such organisms. Previously, medications, nostrums, physics, philtres, and other remedies had been derived from chemical, animal and vegetable matter. Now a new and important word could be admitted to the formularies and the dictionaries *ANTIBIOTIC.*

A new era in medicine had been entered.

And, just as VD had been neglected when the transmission

of infectious diseases was recognized, it was again ignored when this new medical discovery was being put to use to halt other infections. Nothing of a practical nature was done until just before the Japanese bombing of Pearl Harbor, when an American doctor, John F. Mahoney, working on a scientific hunch decided to use penicillin in the treatment of syphilis. He treated four men with early syphilis by giving them injections of penicillin. Three of them became seronegative, and the fourth, while exhibiting no clinical manifestations, retained the positive serology.

Finally, the entering wedge for the management of the syphilis structure had been driven into its very foundation. Fortunately, the discovery came soon after the beginning of World War II. In modern armies, as in the older ones, the most destructive diseases were syphilis and gonorrhea as well as pneumonia. Modern sanitary methods, therapeutics, and immunizations for the different diseases had banished yellow fever, malaria, typhus, and others, but syphilis, gonorrhea and pneumonia remained the greatest health threats to military efficiency; all were controlled by the invention of penicillin.

The manufacture of penicillin was limited to small quantities, and the armed forces made use of all that was available. It saved the Allied armies in the European theater of operations. The camp-followers accompanying the embattled armies were diseased almost to a woman, many of them having both syphilis and gonorrhea. Since prophylactic measures were not as rigidly enforced as they had been during World War I but merely advocated for use, the amount of VD in the invading armies was extremely high. Had it not been for penicillin, the manpower of the onrushing armies would have been greatly depleted.

Eventually, the most ignorant soldier learned that penicillin was a specific for syphilis and gonorrhea. Many soldiers contracted gonorrhea time after time, and syphilis more than once, safe in the thought that all they had to do was get a few injections of penicillin and all would be well!

It was a great day. The age of darkness was being obliterated by the bright lights of science, intelligence, compassion. Man did have a genuine love for his fellow man. And man could pursue his sexual desires and love without fear of contracting or spreading the dread diseases which had previously destroyed him. *VD had been conquered!* Doctors and patients alike thought that syphilis and gonorrhea—those inseparable specters of man's past—had finally been destroyed by man's scientific genius.

Following the war, Public Health Services in the United States established clinics throughout the country. Patients with VD were admitted as in-patients to these "rapid treatment centers" where they were administered an intensive round of penicillin lasting fourteen days. At first, there were a great number of patients, then the numbers began to diminish until, within three to five years, many of these government-institution doors closed for lack of patients.

It was a miracle produced by a miracle drug, penicillin. The fifties marked an era of benign contentment and relaxation in our sexual lives. It was rare that a medical student saw a *chancre* (the initial sore of syphilis) or a well-erupted case of syphilis. There still existed old cases of paresis, tabes dorsalis, gummas, and congenital syphilis—for teaching purposes—but those diseases were the end result of syphilitic infection, which, supposedly, had now been eradicated. Overnight, the syphilologist became the highly respectable dermatologist coping with diseases of the skin, many of which were harmless imitators of the old contagious and horrendous "pox."

The old "red dog" was thought, at last, to be laid to rest.

Then, like a Frankensteinian monster, VD began to emerge anew. First, gonorrhea appeared to be developing a resistance to the miracle drug. Dosages were having to be increased, and the "miraculous" cures were not quite so spectacular. Next, cases of congenital syphilis among newborns were being reported to an extent that doctors began to wonder if the drug had really eliminated syphilis in many of the cases which had been reported "cured." In addition, late syphilitic symptoms began to appear in patients who had been declared cured twenty years earlier. Since the disease was purportedly under control and doctors had relegated it to the research area of disease, a whole new concept of syphilis had to be inaugurated. A bewildered public had to be reeducated. In addition, many doctors had to be trained in the recognition and treatment of the disease when it became apparent that syphilis was again on the rise and very shortly would be out of control.

What had happened?

Why had penicillin failed?

Why VD?

The answers are to be found in the study of venereal disease and its relation to mankind. Three apparent and immediate answers are available:

One: The sexual revolution that followed World War II, and was greatly abetted by the discovery of the "pill"—the oral contraceptive to eliminate unwanted pregnancies—consequently making sexual contacts for women easier and less complicated. The "pill" also caused men to be less careful in the use of prophylaxis—notably the condom, or rubber sheath, which had originally been used for the prevention of disease rather than a means of birth control.

The other feature of the sexual revolution was the open recognition of homosexual activities in what has always been a predominantly heterosexual society. Such organizations as the gay liberation movement forced public recognition and acceptance of sexual practices that had previously, for the most part, been concealed.

Two: The technological, economic, and social changes of the post-war era.

Three: An unfounded confidence in antibiotics, coupled with an apparent negligence in medical research, and public ignorance that resulted in an inability to cooperate in the control and eventual eradication of venereal disease.

When I first undertook the project of writing a book on the subject of VD, I emerged from my role of dermatologist-syphilologist and became something of a roving reporter querying my friends and even casual acquaintances regarding VD. Many people I encountered were unaware that the study of syphilis was the major concern of my specialized field of medicine. They thought of me as a *skin* doctor. When I showed them my credentials, they revealed both to themselves and to me, the ignorance of the public at large concerning VD. I was, frankly, somewhat disquieted with the information I gathered, considering that we live in an era when nude films, topless and bottomless bars, movies depicting all forms of abnormal sexual activity, homosexual and heterosexual, and pornographic literature are easily available, to discover that my customarily garrulous acquaintances were suddenly speechless on the subject of VD.

One fellow doctor conjectured that penicillin, with its short-term cure, had increased promiscuity due to the fact that it had eliminated the long and arduous treatment of the old arsenical and bismuth era. Penicillin, he argued, would never eradicate VD because no disease in the history of medicine had ever been treated out of existence. This part of his argument was correct. The failure of penicillin to help control and eradicate VD was not the failure of the medication. It was man's failure to recognize that penicillin was but a single step in an involved design. To date, man has not developed an immunity to VD, nor has science developed a satisfactory vaccine. This is why it is important that each individual know the entire story of VD. I suppose I should not have been surprised that some vestige of the idea that VD and Divine Punishment was still in existence, but it seemed preposterous for a modern practicing doctor to suggest that the pre-penicillin treatment had the virtue of being so painful that it was sufficiently punitive to make the patient realize that he had to pay the price of torture for his libidinous indiscretions. It seems a morbidly benighted posture.

I then asked one of my friends who had several sons (the youngest is twelve years of age) how he had handled the subject of VD with his children.

He hedged for a moment and then confessed: "I didn't. . . . They learned about it in school. They teach it nowadays." He added, grinning sharply. "Even the little kid knows about VD and what it's all about."

"How do you know?" I asked, innocently.

"He told me," he seemed rather proud and expansive as he continued, "I was walking with him one day and I said, 'Son, do you know what VD means?' He didn't answer for a minute and then he said, 'Sure, Pop, I know what it means.' "

"Did he?" I questioned.

"How the hell do I know? The kid shut up like a clam and I sure as hell wasn't going to pursue the subject. Besides, what the devil would I have told him?"

What, indeed?

2

SYPHILIS IS NOT A DIRTY WORD

Know syphilis in all its forms and manifestations and all other things clinical will be added unto you.
—William Osler, M.D.

The word *syphilis* first appeared in the vocabulary of man in the year 1530 in the poem *Syphilis Sive Morbus Gallicus.* Syphilis was not then the name of the dread venereal disease, but the name of an imaginary shepherd created by one Hieronymous Fracastorius (Girolamo Fracastoro).

Dr. Osler translated Fracastoro's story of the origin of the French disease.

> There is told the story of the discovery of the New World by Columbus and the joy of sailors in its wonders. Unhappily they shot some of the beautiful birds, beloved of the Sun-God, and a prophecy of dire ill was uttered by one of the birds as it escaped:

Nor end your sufferings here; a strange disease,
And most obscene on your bodies seize.

By chance, before they left the natives held a great festival to the Sun-God, but grief was on all faces—"all languished with the same obscene disease," but the priest in snowy robes displayed the boughs of healing guaiacum with which he purged the tainted ground. This the native prince assured the Spanish General was the disease the holy bird had predicted would attack his men, and he told the story of the plague and the discovery of guaiacum as a cure.

A shepherd once (distrust not ancient fame)
Possest these downs and Syphilus was his name.

Syphilus kept the flocks of King Alcithous, and one year the drought was so extreme that the cattle perished for want of water. So incensed was Syphilus that he blasphemed the Sun-God in good terms and decided henceforth to offer no sacrifices to him but to worship King Alcithous. The shepherd won all the people to his way, and the King was overjoyed and proclaimed himself "in earth's sphere to be the only and sufficient diety." But, the Sun-God, enraged, darted forth infection on air, earth, and streams and Syphilus became the first victim of a new disease.

He first wore buboes dreadful to the sight,
First felt strange pains and sleepless
 past the night;
From him the malady received its name.

Becoming a general pestilence, the Sun-God was appealed to and after the proper sacrifices had been made guaiacum was given as a cure for the disease.

This classic poem of Fracastoro was written after Ruy Diaz de Islas published his treatise in which he intimated that he treated some sailors returning from America with Columbus. Although this theory of the origin of syphilis in Europe is no longer accepted as true, this story provides the strongest proof of the American origin of the disease. Many sailors from the Columbian expedition were diseased but young, and the disease was in a latent stage, so it would only be natural for them to travel all over Europe enjoying the praise and adulation of the public. Human beings then were not much different from human beings today and we can compare the excitement and ovations that welcomed the discoverers of a new land beyond the horizon with our own excitement over the space voyages and the kudos lavished upon our astronaut heroes. The sailors were catered to by men eager to hear their tales of adventure and sought after by women who hero-worshipped them. Since the "new" as yet unnamed disease was highly infectious and spread by geometrical progression, it would be not at all impossible for it to have spread over the length and breadth of Europe through the sailors' contacts.

The epidemiology was noted by numerous physicians, and laymen, and especially by the clergy who saw the disease as a manifestation of God's anger and of the punishment of man for his sins. Men with *bösen Blattern* (the evil pox) were prohibited from entering barbershops or public institutions in nearly all the leading cities of the continent. Posters warned men against cohabitating with prostitutes, and the prostitutes, when they were discovered to have the disease, were thrown into jail and retained there until they were either cured or they died. It was not known at this time that syphilis had latent stages when the victims showed no evidence of the disease, but, still infected, were turned loose upon the public. So syphilis, like the floodwaters of the mighty Mississippi, rolled forth over the land contaminating everyone it touched.

The sailors traveled to Barcelona, where their majesties King Ferdinand and Queen Isabella were in residence, and the town was resplendent in their honor. But the sailors, who were apparently at this time quite healthy, decided to move on to Italy, to Rome and to Naples, where they arrived in the early spring of 1494, leaving in their wake memories of their visit in scourges of the new disease.

In December 1494 King Charles VIII crossed the Alps to besiege Naples. His army was composed of mercenaries and soldiers of fortune from practically every country in Europe, including Russia. In his book entitled *The Serpentine Disease,* Juan de Vigo, private physician to the Pope, wrote:

> Afterwards in the following year 1494, the most Catholic King Charles of France, who was then reigning, having guided a great army, passed into Italy and at the time he entered the country with his host many Spaniards infected with the disease were in it and at once the camp began to be infected by this malady and the French who did not know what it was thought that it came from the atmosphere in the region. The French called it The Disease of Naples and the Italians and Neapolitans called it The French Disease.
>
> From that time on as it continued to spread they gave it a name each one according to his opinion as to how the disease had its origin. I called it the *Serpentine Disease of the Island of Española* because according to its loathesomeness I do not know anything to which I could more naturally compare it than to the serpent. Whereas a serpent is ugly, fearful and horrid, so is this disease ugly, fearful and horrid. A grave disease that separates and corrupts the flesh and breaks and rots the

> bones and disrupts and contracts the nerves, and consequently I gave it that name.

The Columbian theory is as controversial today as it was in the fifteenth century. Some scholars point to evidence of syphilis found in bones which predate Columbus's journey, and other scholars feel there is some foundation for the belief that the leprosy referred to in biblical writings and in other early histories was, as a matter of fact, syphilis. These arguments are not unlike the arguments over Shakespeare and Sir Francis Bacon as to who really wrote the Shakespearean plays. And does it really matter except as a scholarly exercise?

The original source of syphilis is as much a mystery today as it was when it was first witnessed. It is thanks to the writing of Fracastoro that modern medicine owes much of its knowledge of the course the disease, and as well its eventual name, syphilis. From the time of its recognition, syphilis has been pursued by a portentous mass of confused literature. Alarm, misunderstanding, religious emotion, false modesty, willful misrepresentation, and the change in the type of the disease itself have all contributed much mythology to a naturally difficult subject. Fracastoro accomplished a mammoth undertaking by bringing some order out of the confusion.

One scholar, Dr. Frédéric Buret of Paris, tracing the history of syphilis in 1889, presents a reasonably argued case that syphilis was known to ancient China and Japan, to the Hebrews, the Hindus, the Greeks, and the Romans, continuing to appear in Europe through the Middle Ages and down the years preceding the voyage of Columbus. Both its venereal and congenital aspects were recognized from the beginning. There are records from the third millennium B.C. of the separation of the syphilitic chancre from the one that is known today as the soft chancre or *chancroid*, of both from gonorrhea, and of the use of mercury for treatment!

Since the origin of syphilis is quite debatable, we must

delve into the nature and characteristics of the disease itself. The relationship of the diagnosis and management of syphilis has become inverted in the past generation. Once, cases of infectious syphilis were common and easy to diagnose, but their treatment was difficult. An expert was required to cope with reactions to arsenic and bismuth, and nothing short of a silver-tongued orator like William Jennings Bryan or a golden-boy Billy Graham could persuade a patient of the necessity of completing the long-term treatment.

Today lesion syphilis is less common. Thanks to penicillin, therapy is simple, but diagnosis has become complicated. More and more persons are receiving penicillin or another treponemicidal antibiotics for so many reasons that the signs and symptoms of early syphilis are often suppressed or modified, and the serologic reactions are atypical.

Syphilis—the love sickness—is thought to have begun as a disease of cities and the sexual sophistication which is more common to cities than to rural life. The truly suitable contact for the syphilis spirochete is sexual intercourse. Since the spirochetes grow well in the genital area and produce sores there, genital transfer is a logical mode of transportation for them.

Syphilis is a slow disease as microbial diseases go. The spirochetes have been found to divide in two every thirty hours as compared to every twenty or thirty minutes for most disease bacteria. They probably penetrate through a break in the skin on a moist surface, but the tiniest scratch is enough. It is estimated that several hundred spirochetes are usually present during the transmitting event. Some of them fail to get through and die in the attempt, and, depending on the stage of the disease in its source—in terms of relative developing immunity—some may not survive after they get through. But when the infection comes from early active disease in which there is no immunity or only a trace of it, all the spirochetes that get in may multiply and keep on doing so. This is the highest degree of infectiousness we know.

In venereal syphilis, there is likely to develop at the point of inoculation—nearly always on the penis or somewhere in the region of the vulva or the vagina—a single sore called a chancre or a *hard chancre.* "Hard" refers to the circle of rubbery tissue around the base of the sore, and is contrasted with the similar but "soft" chancre of the minor venereal disease called "chancroid." The primary sore of syphilis is nearly always single and painless. It grows over a period of days or a week or more from a small pimple to a sore the size of a marble, and tends to break down on top and form an ulcer. The lymph nodes in the area, usually the groin, become large and hard. Spirochetes are present in the fluid that can be squeezed out of the chancre. They are also in the lymph nodes. Found under these conditions, they establish the diagnosis of syphilis.

The chancre is peculiar to syphilis and it only appears in the primary stage . . . and *sometimes it does not appear at all.* In fact, if one has contacted syphilis, one is fortunate if a chancre appears and medical attention can be procured immediately. The chancre heals of itself and as it does, or some time later, a rash appears on the body—all over or on any part of it—including the skin of the palms of the hands and the soles of the feet, in the mouth as well as around the genitalia and the anus. This is the secondary stage. In syphilis, these lesions are usually painless, seldom itch, and are not destructive; that is they heal with or without treatment with little or no scarring. A person who does not suspect what they are may pass off the lesions without attaching any significance to them.

Pain and discomfort are not always absent in secondary syphilis. There is often a very sore throat and hoarseness. Headaches may occur. There may be pain in the bones and joints, very often only at night. In more severe cases there may be a patchy loss of hair from the head or the eyebrows and eyelashes. And there is a rare malignant form of syphilis which may be the deadly form of the disease of the fifteenth century. Large ugly sores on the skin and the moist surfaces ulcerate and form scabs or crusts. If these should attack the vital organs, death follows.

In the normal, unattended course of the disease, the spirochetes multiply in the lymph nodes that drain the spot where the first chancre appears, and spill over into the blood. Once they reach the bloodstream, the microbes are carried all over the body. They settle out at the ends of the capillaries and grow again, leading to irritation and damage as their numbers reach a high enough level. These generalized lesions may show themselves while the chancre is still present or while it heals, or some time may intervene without symptoms; as many as six months may pass before new lesions appear. These lesions and symptoms tend to heal and disappear again, leaving no trace.

Late symptoms appear after another variable interval of "silent infection" or latency which may last as long as twenty years. These late lesions involve the blood vessels and the heart, the eyes, and parts of the central nervous system. The resulting destruction of tissue and associated symptoms in the cardiovascular or nervous systems or the eye cannot be treated successfully, although the process may be arrested at any time. Neurosyphilis includes the two patterns called respectively "tabes" (tabes dorsalis—also called locomotor ataxia—is syphilis of the spinal cord characterized especially by a peculiar, halting gait), and "general paresis" (dementia paralytica, general paralysis of the insane)—syphilis of the brain itself.

Congenital syphilis, meaning an infection passing through the placenta from the syphilitic mother to the fetus in the womb so that the baby is born with the disease, is most likely to happen if the mother has infectious syphilis after the fourth month of pregnancy. Depending upon the severity of the case, it may lead to a miscarriage at any time after the fourth month, to a baby stillborn at the regular term, or to one born alive with syphilis. In such a baby, syphilis is already generalized and the symptoms can be secondary or tertiary or both together. Characteristically, there may be a destructive ulcer of the bridge of the nose so that it falls in (saddle nose), blindness from opacity of the cornea, and peculiarly shaped permanent teeth, especially the upper incisors, the sides of which curve inward toward the biting edge, the edge itself being notched, and strawberry molars, so-called because of their appearance. An associated symptom is deafness due to syphilis of the auditory nerve. These three defects are known as Hutchinson's triad, after Sir Jonathan Hutchinson who discovered them in 1859.

Congenital syphilis includes many varieties. The newborn infant may appear healthy or may have no more than the sore mouth or throat of secondary syphilis. The congenital syphilitic who survives may die from a cardiovascular accident or a lesion in some other vital spot, or may live on with more or less deformity. Bony deformities are most common, including protruding brows and abnormalities of the upper jaw, as well as a saddle nose. "Saber shins," a forward bowing of the leg bones, is a familiar condition.

The most important step in syphilis is proper diagnosis and early treatment. Most people are alerted to an annual physical check-up, but if a person knows or suspects that he has been exposed to syphilis and can see any of the signs herein described—a sore on the genitals, a skin rash not definitely explained in other terms—he should go posthaste to a qualified physician or a VD clinic.

In the chancre stage of syphilis, diagnosis depends on identifying spirochetes in the sore or, sometimes, in the regional lymph nodes. The best way to do this is with a darkfield microscope, which means that the patient and the microscope are not too far apart. Given the equipment and the necessary skill, the test can be made in a few minutes. Failure to identify the organism from a suspect lesion by darkfield examination may mean that: 1) the lesion is not syphilitic; 2) the patient has received antisyphilitic drugs locally or systematically; 3) too much time has elapsed since the appearance of the lesion; 4) the lesion may be of late syphilis; 5) further examination might be required.

The expert can usually distinguish *Treponema pallidum* from the nonpathogenic spirochetes occurring in the genital or skin lesions. However, normal spirochetes from the mouth or the anus can be confused with *T. pallidum.* If the physician takes the fluid from a lymph node or a dry sore, the chances of error are small. A positive darkfield with appropriate clinical signs and history justify starting treatment at once.

The darkfield test can be used on the rash of early infectious syphilis, but by the time the rash has appeared antibodies have usually been formed and tests on blood for their presence become the basis of syphilis diagnosis.

There are several different groups of blood tests for syphilis. The first, and most familiar to the layman, is the Wasserman test, which was discovered by Wasserman and his team in 1906. The test is based on an antibody which has no direct connection with the spirochete of syphilis. A more recent group of tests became available in 1949. They are based directly on an antibody to *Treponema pallidum.* The original and key member of the group is the *Treponema pallidum* immobilization *(TPI)* test. Spirochetes for the test are taken from an infected rabbit and injected into the testicles of healthy rabbits, where they multiply so abundantly that in a week or so the testicles are much enlarged and full of active, virulent spirochetes. This, incidentally, is the closest that science has come to a culture method for the spirochete of syphilis. In another group, we find a single test dating from 1957 based on a noninfectious spirochete called the *Reiter treponeme,* which can be grown in ordinary culture and is therefore more easily obtainable in larger quantity.

The reliability of these tests is measured in terms of *sensitivity* and *specificity.* A test can show negative even though the patient has syphilis, and it may show positive even when the patient doesn't have the disease. A sensitive test picks up more cases of syphilis, misses fewer, and does not turn up as many false negatives. A specific test tends to be positive only in syphilis; it shows fewer false positives.

At the Venereal Disease Research Laboratories in Atlanta, Georgia, a simpler test was worked out which is known by the initials of the laboratory *VDRL.* It is one of the most widely used for premarital screening, preliminary tests, and tests done routinely for private physicians, and is coming into use all over the world. The RPR or *rapid plasma reagin* test was perfected in 1962 and designed for rapid screening under field conditions. It is especially useful in testing migrant workers and people on the move. If a positive reaction is found in the RPR test, blood can then be tested by one of the more standard, more specific, tests.

If clinical indications and history point to syphilis, a negative test naturally gives rise to suspicion and a repeat test is required. A positive test in the absence of history or clinical signs causes the most agony for a patient. Some false positives are biologic—meaning that some substance is present in the blood that causes the reaction, but false in the sense that syphilis is absent.

All these tests are a definite aid in the diagnosis of syphilis, and they are used as almost the sole basis for the diagnosis of latent syphilis.

The only completely satisfactory means of diagnosing neurosyphilis accurately and of evaluating its treatment properly is by spinal-fluid examinations. With the introduction of penicillin and other antibiotics, the need for spinal-fluid examinations in the management of syphilitic patients is no longer quite as important as when treatment was confined to arsenic and bismuth therapy. It was essential to diagnose the condition because it required special therapy, and the treatment with arsenic and bismuth failed to arrest neurosyphilis satisfactorily in many cases. Penicillin is now the treatment of choice for all types of syphilis, and is usually capable of arresting permanently all types of neurosyphilis. Consequently, spinal-fluid examinations of syphilitics are no longer quite as essential as formerly.

The treatment of syphilis by penicillin can be sufficient for any stage of the disease if adequate blood levels are maintained for a sufficient time. The penicillin can be the short or the long-acting, "depot," type. It may be suspended in an aluminum salt and may contain a local anesthetic. Injections of penicillin are preferable to oral medication, since absorption is highly variable, and patient cooperation in taking the entire treatment is not always obtained.

When penicillin sensitivity precludes the use of this drug of choice, some of the newer antibiotics are the best alternatives. Recommended dosage for erythromycin and tetracycline is 20 to 30 grams given over a period of 10 to 15 days. Treatments with such alternate antibiotics must be accompanied by a close follow-up of the syphilitic patient, since none of these drugs has had adequate evaluation in all stages of syphilis. Spinal-fluid examinations should be done routinely as part of the follow-up after this type of therapy.

Treatment of a syphilitic patient, particularly in an early stage, without examining his or her contacts, contributes very little to the overall control of the disease. If treatment were confined only to obviously infected persons who volunteered for diagnosis and treatment, neither warnings nor the necessary medical aid could be administered to the syphilitic patient's contacts, making any control of syphilis impossible.

Every sex contact to infectious syphilis should be located, examined, and evaluated for possible treatment. Treatment should be administered either on the basis of the treatment of diagnosed infected individuals, or on the basis of preventive or prophylactic treatment of all persons who have been exposed sexually to infectious syphilis and who, although negative on physical and serologic examination, may be in the incubation period or may have small undetected primary lesions.

If the reader is truly concerned, it should be stated that anyone known to have been exposed to lesion syphilis is extremely foolish to wait for the disease to develop to the clinical or reactive serologic stage, meanwhile allowing re-infection of treated patients and the infection of additional victims.

It is under rare circumstances that a patient with primary or secondary syphilis may have had no additional contact since the beginning of his or her incubation period, because most people who get infected lead a rather promiscuous sex life and tend to associate with persons who do the same thing. Usually, when two individuals name each other as the reciprocal contacts, it is not from one another that they contracted syphilis. There must be at least one other infected individual. In addition to his or her source of infection the average syphilis patient may be expected to name three or four other contacts; and it is not rare for infected patients to name from 20 to as many as 70 contacts in a 3 to 6 month period. Any one of these contacts not located and examined may develop the disease, pass it on to other persons, and become afflicted later with damaging manifestations.

Primary syphilis patients should be interviewed for all contacts going back to three months prior to the manifestations which have brought the patient to a doctor. Secondary patients should be interviewed going back six months prior to the onset of symptoms. Early latent syphilis patients should be interviewed going back to at least one year.

Interviewing patients and tracing their contacts requires considerable skill and time. Unless the patient is highly co-operative, the time required is often beyond the ability of the private physician to give. However, most health departments are able and anxious to provide the epidemologic services to private physicians

Before ending the chapter on syphilis—the top banana of VD—it might be an excellent idea to let the reader comprehend just how fortunate (despite the current epidemic identity of VD) that he or she is a contemporary suffering from a disease for which there is a specific. Some of the cures of the past seem, even to a venereologist, to be inappropriate, and begin to assume a sadistic identity while the victim comes off smelling like a masochist. Let us take a quick look at the pre-penicillin treatments for syphilis.

For three centuries before the introduction of Salvarsan (606, or the *silver bullet*) most syphilologists used mercury and the iodides, or their combination, by mouth. In the nineteenth century, injections of the solution of bichloride of mercury were given as often as twice a day in a malignant case. One course of treatment consisted of twenty injections. Good results were claimed, but the mercurial injections were discontinued because of the pain to the patient, abscesses, severe grades of salivation, and other manifestations of mercury poisoning that were produced. The popular quotation then was, "one night with Venus and the rest of your life with Mercury." Actually, under the bright light of modern medicine mercury is thought to have had little effect upon any type of syphilis except late syphilis. The therapeutics of syphilis in the days when there were few specific remedies was truly an array of the most amazing drugs, and everything the doctors could think of was used—from the infusion of holy wood to the giving of animal excretions and a whole galaxy of minerals.

One of the groups of chemicals that were utilized after the work of William Wallace were the iodides, particularly useful in the late manifestations of the disease. Although not a spirocheticide, potassium iodide, used empirically, helped remarkably to cure those patients with advanced stages of syphilis. Before that time clinics all over the world were replete with revolting scenes, patients with great indolent ulcers that exposed the bones and noseless faces emitting powerful fetid breaths.

Obviously, when man is on the search for a "superkiller," and discoveries in bacteriological areas advance to a stage that diagnostic methods are almost perfected (or at least brought to such a degree of development that millions of new cases of syphilis can be discovered) it is only logical that a better method for the treatment of the disease would be developed.

In 1908, a German chemist, Dr. Paul Erlich, began the research which ended with the production of Salvarsan, one of the family of arsphenamines, as they are called today. Dr. Erlich knew that arsenic had been used in the treatment of the disease since treatment was first recorded. With a Japanese assistant, Hata, he began to build arsenical organic compounds with the benzene ring as a base. His laboratory was well supplied with rats which were inoculated with a type of trypanosome which was susceptible to arsenical compounds.

Erlich and Hata patiently made and remade many batches, and experimented with thousands of rats. In most cases, the arsenical compound would kill the parasite but would also kill the rat! Finally, on the *606th try,* Erlich succeeded in *killing the organism without killing the rat.*

The law of therapeutic index which Lister had established was confirmed. Erlich called the product *SALVARSAN*—"Arsenic saves."

The dosage obviously had to be examined by trial and error, first in rats, then in human beings. The arsenic compound was dissolved in distilled water and later neutralized with sodium hydroxide until the cloudy solution was cleared. If the unneutralized solution was given, as it was in some cases, the patient died. Finally about 20cc of the arsenical solution were used. It was drawn off into the 10cc syringes and the contents were injected under the shoulder blades or into the buttocks. The result was miraculous. Spirochetes disappeared from the primary lesion within twenty-four hours and secondary eruptions began to disappear in a few days. Clinics for the treatment commenced to spring up all over the world, for the treatment was a hospital procedure. Unfortunately, many patients died of the treatment rather than the disease and, despite this "wonder treatment," the course of syphilis was not going well.

Under the direction of Surgeon General Dr. Thomas Parran and the United States Public Health Service, a rational treatment program was established. It was determined that seventy-two weeks of continuous treatment was adequate therapy. It was found that this method, which consisted of alternate courses of arsphenamine and bismuth, would cure approximately 75 percent of the early syphilitics, a lesser number of those with late syphilis and late, latent syphilis, and a still smaller degree of the older syphilitics.

It was not until 1917 that Julius Wagner-Jauregg, a Viennese psychiatrist, devised a method of efficient treatment of late syphilis to replace the horrendous earlier methods. He conceived the idea of inoculating his patients (paretics) with *benign tertian malaria.* He did this because he noted earlier that paretics who were accidentally inoculated with malaria often had remissions and, in some, the remissions seemed to be permanent. The first case upon whom he used it reacted very favorably and lived for many years in an apparently healthy state.

Malarial therapy became a favorite and was used by nearly all the syphilologists in the world. The malarial treatment of paretics was a standard treatment in nearly all the institutions for the insane. It was also necessary to hospitalize persons with less severe manifestations of syphilis because of the dangers that attended this method of treatment. Age was a great determining factor, and it was with hesitation that a man over fifty years of age was inoculated with this malaria remedy.

It is of interest to the student of syphilis to note that Ruy

Diaz de Islas (see chapter 1) observed the beneficial effects of malarial disease upon the syphilitic four hundred years before Wagner-Jauregg used this method of treatment.

When malaria was used, every patient had to be hospitalized for as long as six weeks, for it was estimated that forty hours of temperature about 104 degrees was minimum adequate treatment. While malarial treatment was the best type of treatment that had ever been used in the control of paresis until then, therapists were constantly on the lookout for new methods. No one could decide whether it was some agent in the body of the malarial parasite or in the human cells that was responsible. After due consideration many scientists came to believe that it was the fever that was the main factor responsible for the good results.

The realization of this fact led them to induce temperature fever by artificial means, first by the use of diathermy, a treatment that originated in the twenties and from which good results were obtained, and next, by the use of the heat box in which infrared heat rays were used to bring about a rise in temperature. This was quite a dangerous process, for the patient was likely to suffer either from a heat stroke or from heat exhaustion. In many ways it was more dangerous than the malarial treatment, and the same contraindications were present; there were a number of deaths due to side reactions. Then came the electronic cabinet of Kettering, originally constructed to treat rheumatic ailments, which produced high temperatures within the body, while the temperature within the cabinet did not rise about 112 degrees Farenheit. The results, however, were not as satisfactory as those produced by malarial inoculation.

The problems presented by the heat box and malarial inoculation were that many institutions could not afford the former nor could they procure malaria for inoculation. Some other method had to be devised. The utilization of the hot bath was that method. In the last decade of the fifteenth century the hot bath was used by Francisco Lopéz de Villalobos, and he recorded good results from it in the treatment of paretics. It was in the 20s that it was discovered that this treatment by hot baths was effective in raising the body's resistance to late syphilis. It was a remarkable thing that the syphilitic manifestations which would not resolve after the use of arsphenamines, bismuth, and mercury would respond to the use of hot baths. The patient was placed in a tub of water at body temperature and the heat raised rapidly to 112 degrees or 115 degrees. There was a sharp rise in body temperature to as high as 105 or 106 degrees.

It was thought this specific treatment would be more effective if mapharsen was given intravenously at the height of the induced temperature. The arsenicals could not be given to patients being treated with malaria because of the fear that in conjunction with arsenic it might prove fatal. Often the patient was swathed in a heat-controlled blanket and administered mapharsen at the same time. But all those methods of treatment were fraught with dangers, and occasionally, death. When it became recognized that heat was an important part of the "cure," the spas were crowded—notably, Hot Springs, Arkansas, in the United States—where affluent and prominent syphilitics basked in the heat of the natural springs and forgot their maladies temporarily in the excitement of the nearby racetrack and the illegal gambling casinos. Among the more notorious patrons of the Springs' therapeutic baths was the gangster, Al Capone, who eventually died of paresis while interned on the "Rock" at Alcatraz.

In the twenties, the entire world was eager to find a specific cure for one of man's most insidious and dread diseases. Hope was generated when the spirochete which was the cause of the disease was identified, and sundry medications appeared that promised miracle cures for its conquest, only to be extinguished when the wiggly killer was found to have been lying dormant for fifteen to twenty years before reappearing in the final virulent stage of its crippling or killing role. Men and women who had thought themselves cured, who married and had children during the noninfectious period, awoke to the true horrors of syphilis. It did, indeed, seem to be a ravaging, relentless blow dealt to mankind by a maleficent fate. The victims cringed in their fear and in the inability of medicine to solve the problem. In their hour of doom, they heard the ominous voice echoing from above, reminding them of the curse rendered unto those iniquitous ones "unto the third and fourth generation"!

It was at the time when the recognition of the hopelessness of finding a cure was most prevalent that penicillin was discovered by Fleming. It was greeted with a deep sigh of relief: VD and all of its attendant horrors would be eradicated within two generations. But it was not to be so easy. The crafty spirillum had outsmarted the enemy agents by hiding in the medical Trojan horses—content to lie quiet until the proper time came when they would rise again to baffle patient and doctor alike.

Any treated syphilitic may, at a later date, need additional treatment. This should be noted especially by those people who contracted syphilis a generation ago and have rested content in the belief that the disease was eliminated. There are four conditions in which additional treatment is indicated: 1) syphilis in pregnancy when adequacy of previous treatment is not determinable; 2) persistently active neurosyphilis; 3) relapse; and 4) reinfection.

In pregnancy, when there is a possible doubt as to the mother's having been adequately treated or any suspicion of an active infection, a course of therapy should be administered for the prevention of congenital syphilis in the child. The amount of penicillin with which the mother should be treated should be governed by her diagnosis and her body's acceptance of the drug.

In neurosyphilis, if the cell count of the spinal fluid does not return to normal within one year, or if there is an increase in cells or protein during the follow-up period, retreatment is indicated. As a rule, the amount of penicillin for treatment need not exceed 10 million units.

Relapse, or reinfection. It is often difficult to determine in a given case whether one is confronted by a relapse or a reinfection. The principal significance of such a decision lies in the fact that a reinfection is treated exactly as a new case, whereas a relapse may require increased antibiotic therapy or retreatment, if a low dosage schedule was initially used. Treatment relapses are much less common than formerly assumed, most cases so diagnosed actually being reinfections.

In early syphilis, the concentration of circulating antibodies descends rapidly and regularly after treatment if therapy has been adequate and prompt. Failure of therapy or a rise in titer may herald either a relapse or a reinfection.

A reinfection is often indicated by a new primary lesion at a site different from the last primary lesion, a serology suggestive of a new infection, and a history of exposure.

Because of previous sensitization to the *T. pallidum*, reinfections may produce skin and mucous membrane lesions approaching, morphologically and histologically, those of the manifestations of late benign syphilis, suggesting late relapse rather than reinfection. However, the ease of darkfield demonstration of *T. pallida*, plus history, should be sufficient to establish reinfection.

Relapse or sero-fastness? If syphilis remains untreated for a number of years, the serologic titer often becomes fixed. No amount of treatment will alter this appreciably. This does not mean that the patient needs retreatment. It generally indicates a "burnt-out" infection. Retreatment is indicated only in the presence of persistent abnormal cell count and protein in the spinal fluid or of a persistent rise in serologic titer.

In the days prior to penicillin and antibiotics, there existed a sort of lengthy limerick which was used quite aptly to illustrate the course of syphilis to young medical students. I quote it here as a bit of levity to be added to the serious aspect of syphilis from beginning to end. Although humorous, it is accurate, and illustrates the invincibility of the disease and the ultimate fate of its victims.

There was a young man from Back Bay
Who thought syphilis just went away.
  He believed that a chancre
  Was only a canker
That healed in a week and a day.

But now he has *acne vulgaris*
(Or whatever they call it in Paris)
  On his skin it has spread
  From his feet to his head,
And his friends want to know where his hair is.

There's more to his terrible plight;
His pupils won't close in the light
  His heart is cavorting,
  His wife is aborting,
And he squints through his gun-barrel sight.

Arthralga cuts into his slumber
His aorta's in need of a plumber;
  By now he has tabes,
  And saber-shinned babies,
While of gummas he's got quite a number.

He's been treated in every known way,
His spirochetes grow day by day;
  He's developed paresis
  Has long talks with Jesus
And thinks he's the Queen of the May!

ANONYMOUS

3

GONORRHEA: A DOSE OF CLAP?

In the story of VD, syphilis and gonorrhea are the handmaidens of diseases contracted through sexual contact. Where syphilis has always had the element of fear associated with its progress and had an early and marked association with insanity, death, and congenital effects, gonorrhea for many years was taken more lightly, thought of as a "cold" or a "strain." In fact, among certain cultures, it was almost disregarded and treated casually as one of those only-to-be-expected minor accidents encountered along the road to sexual maturity.

Gonorrhea is a contagious disease of the greatest importance because of its widespread and constant presence in the human race in every part of the world. It is a menace, not only on account of its extraordinary prevalence, but also because its effects in some individuals may be far-reaching and disastrous. It is well known that gonorrhea is one of the most important causes of blindness in the world. It is the chief cause of sterility in both male and female, and is the cause of at least 50 percent of the total gynecological complaints from which women suffer.

The dangerous and far-reaching effects of gonorrhea are due to the fact that many local complications such as prostatitis, epididymitis, cervicitis, metritritis, salpingitis, and ovaritis are very common. Even metastatic complications in the remotest parts of the body such as arthritis, iritis, endocarditis, etc., are by no means rare.

The serious menace of the disease is further increased because of the great difficulty in curing many cases, and because of the ineluctability of the complaint, more especially in women.

Exact figures on the prevalence and spread of gonorrhea are very difficult to obtain, because it varies to some extent amongst different peoples and different classes of society. Also, it is a disease which the patient tends to keep secret even from his own physician, opting rather to go for treatment to some stranger or to a clinic.

The continual and widespread occurrence of gonorrhea is a "sign of the times." Generations ago, in remote agricultural areas before the development of the steamship, the railroad, the automobile, the airplane, the telephone and telegraph, the disease was not so commonplace, but, like most other infectious diseases, the opportunities for spreading increased with trade and travel, penetrating into the farthermost parts of the world. The continuance of war and the transporting of millions of human beings into distant lands amongst foreign peoples is part of the pattern.

Before the discovery of penicillin, the gonococcus succumbed to sulfonamide action, but during the seven years before penicillin became available, gonococcal strains occasionally developed resistance to concentrations in excess of those tolerated by the host. Just as the moment when hope was waning of ever finding a substitute for the once successful sulfonamides, penicillin burst forth as a seemingly ideal therapeutic agent. Today, however, we have awakened to the realization that, even after having employed the most revolutionary therapeutic agent ever discovered, in combination with vigorous case-finding efforts, we must admit that control of gonorrhea has failed.

Why? Again let us trace the disease and discover the answer.

For such an ancient and pervading disease, advances in knowledge about gonorrhea have come about slowly. While medical historians are not in accord, it is believed by many that the venereal character of the disease was known to the early Jews and described in Leviticus XV. Galen in 130 AD was responsible for the name "gonorrhea," meaning "flow of seed." In the fifth century before Christ, Hippocrates (who also is credited by some medical historians with inventing the name) was certainly cognizant that gonorrhea was infectious and was carried by contact from one person to another. But exact data regarding the antiquity of gonorrhea, its first appearance in the human race, and its mode of spread over the whole world, are unfortunately missing, even though it has been proved beyond doubt that the disease was known to all ancient civilized peoples.

Historically, the record of gonorrhea is confused and always debatable, not only because of early man's ignorance in regard to contagion, but also because diagnosis from ancient descriptions of a disease is a tricky business for the most erudite of diagnosticians. However, there are suggestive references to gonorrhea in ancient Egyptian prescriptions, in early Chinese and Japanese sources, and in Biblical and Vedic writings. In the writings of the legendary Emperor Huang Ti (c. 2698-c. 2597 B.C.) there is this recorded paraphrase of a description which would fit gonorrhea. "Among the external diseases there is one that is different from all others in the symptoms which are easy to recognize: They are 1) affections of the urethra and vagina at the same time as the bladder, 2) drainage of corrupt materials white or red by the urethra or vagina."

Descriptions suggestive of gonorrhea are also found on an ancient Assyrian tablet which speaks of cloudy or thick urine; in Hippocrates there is mention of "strangury" or stricture (blockage) of the urethra, both of which are manifestations of gonorrhea; and there is also foundation for the belief that during the European Dark Ages, Arabian doctors were familiar with the disease. A well-known Persian physician, Rhazes (c. 860-c. 925), would appear to have been as talented as any modern genito-urinary specialist. It is known that he differentiated smallpox from measles; used animal gut for sutures; introduced mercurial ointments; that he wrote a detailed description of strictures and the immediate introduction of a catheter if there was any degree of retention of urine. His other writings include a medical encyclopedia and other works on nervous diseases.

In the history of medicine, it would appear that Avicenna (in Arabic, Ibn Sina, 980-1037 *A.D.*), who is known in the West for his *Canons of Medicine*, was the first physician to use catheters made from the skins of various animals. He also mentions intravesical ("into the bladder") injections by means of a silver syringe. In the thirteenth century, we encounter a William of Saliceto who seemed to have diagnosed gonorrhea and recognized its venereal nature. William attributed the disease to impurities retained under the male prepuce after exposure to an unclean woman. He suggested washing as a method of prevention . . . a suggestion which, harking back to early basic toilet training, is also highly recommended today. Gonorrhea as a venereal disease was known in early England, and we find references to the disease in periodicals and writings of the fourteenth century, where gonorrhea is identified with the words *ardor, arsura,* or *indendium* or by the more recently anglicized words *brenning* or *burning.*

The contagious character was so generally recognized in the Middle Ages that attempts were made to use prophylactic measures to prevent the spread of the disease—measures such as police regulations and the examination of prostitutes. This knowledge was unfortunately almost completely lost when, toward the middle of the fifteenth century, syphilis made its appearance in Europe, and spread, in the Great Epidemic, over all the countries of the old world.

At this time, gonorrhea was identified with syphilis, and was, in fact, regarded by many physicians and laymen as a mild form of syphilis. Knowledge of the diverse identities of gonorrhea and syphilis was further recorded as the result of the unfortunate vaccination experiment of John Hunter (1728-1793), surgeon extraordinary to George III for whom the Hunterian chancre is named. He inoculated himself with the purulent matter from a syphilitic sore on the penis of a rogue condemned to death, and developed both syphilis and gonorrhea. This added greatly to the confusion, until Philippe Ricord (1800-1899), who became the personal physician to Napoleon III, demonstrated, in 1832, by a series of comprehensive experiments that the two diseases were distinct, different, and independent of each other. Fortunately, his work was generally acknowledged, but Ricord, strange to say, although convinced of the contagious character of syphilis, was entirely opposed to the opinion that gonorrhea was of an infectious nature. He maintained that gonorrhea was simply a catarrh of the urethral mucous membrane, caused by a diversity of irritants. He also believed that menstrual, lochial, and puerperal discharges could cause gonorrhea in man by their irritant properties.

Ricord's erroneous belief in the noncontagious character of gonorrhea luckily was soon contradicted. When at last it dawned upon the medical profession that the disease was undoubtedly contagious, efforts were made to discover the causative agent, and many species of organisms were put forward as the specific cause of the malady. This groping in the dark came to an end in 1879, when the German physician Albert Neisser (1855-1916), recognizing the importance of the bacteriological technique of Koch, initiated an investigation of gonorrheal secretions by up-to-date methods—and discovered the *gonococcus.* In his treatise "A New Species of Coccus Specific to Gonorrhea" Neisser described the new organism as being a diplococcus, whose opposing sides were generally flattened out, creating a characteristic coffee-bean shape. He also pointed out the peculiar grouping of the germs within the pus cells and upon the epithelial cells and, further, that these free extracellular forms were usually found in groups of four, eight, twelve, etc., never in chains.

The problem of diagnosing gonorrhea can be as difficult, on occasion, as that of syphilis. If there is pain and pus, the diagnosis of gonorrhea can be arrived at in a matter of minutes, with further confirmation obtainable within twenty-four to forty-eight hours, but, in the case of many women, neither evidence of the disease may be apparent. The same is also true of the infected male homosexual.

An unexpected element in the nationwide gonorrhea epidemic has surfaced recently. The man with asymptomatic gonorrhea may be playing a much larger role in perpetuating the epidemic than either the medical profession or the public has previously suspected. The misconception that all men are symptomatic and all women asymptomatic alters the control aspects of the disease. A recent study conducted by the VD control program of the Norfolk, Virginia, Department of Health reports that 10 to 15 percent—possibly 20 percent—of the male contacts of infected women develop their infections without showing any signs or symptoms, and maintain the asymptomatic state for many weeks—some for as long as 14 weeks—during which time these disease spreaders continue their sexual activity without suspecting that they are infected. The Norfolk study indicates that rectal involvement is probably the result of direct implantation of the gonococcus organism. In women this results from heterosexual contact, and in men, obviously, from homosexual contact. Over 90 percent of the men in the study with rectal gonorrhea admitted to having had homosexual contact.

Similarly, pharyngeal gonorrhea must also be considered a result of oral sexual contact, as it is now the third most common asymptomatic site of involvement. To test the frequency of oral involvement, all gonorrhea patients in the Norfolk VD clinic were asked, during a seven-month period in 1971, whether or not they practiced fellatio. (For general information about fellatio, the reader is referred to the Linda Lovelace movie *Deep Throat.*) Of the 586 patients who were questioned, 138, or 24 percent, said they did indeed practice fellatio. Pharyngeal gonorrhea was found in 31, or 22 percent, of the group. Interestingly enough, of the group of 138, most were female, white, and largely of the middle or upper middle class.

The study raises the question (in view of the fact that many in the group may have practiced fellatio without having admitted to it) whether or not in a really complete routine survey for gonorrhea, the cervix, the rectum, the urethra, and the pharynx should not all be tested. The study certainly reveals that the practice of fellatio is not confined to the homosexual.

If a woman has had only one heterosexual partner (gonorrhea is rarely spread among practicing Lesbians) and she is ignorant of his sexual activities with other men or women, she may never suspect the presence of gonorrhea before it has entered into the pelvis and Fallopian tubes—with irreparable damage. Often chronic pelvic inflammatory disease or complete sterility results. Even when compulsory examinations are made of prisoners and prostitutes, for example, the presence of infection will very often be by-passed.

To make a diagnosis of gonorrhea, a drop of pus is usually examined under a microscope using a glass slide and quite an ordinary stain. The procedure is painless to the patient and usually takes about five minutes. Diagnosis is based upon the appearance of typical paired gonococci inside so-called pus cells (phagocytes). The picture, however, is not always typical and it may be imitated by somewhat similar bacteria that are not gonococci. We can find false negatives and false positives in gonorrhea quite as often as in cases of syphilis.

The customary way to resolve such an ambiguity is to

make a culture of the gonococcus in which it can be identified without further question. The culture grows out in twenty-four hours, and another day may be needed for final identifying tests. The one attendant difficulty in ferreting out the gonococcus lies in its fragility. Modern laboratory facilities have managed to keep the gonococcus culture alive for sufficient lengths of time to diagnose it properly. However, the diagnosis of gonorrhea is often impeded through the lack of a blood test as a means of identification, since it is generally a localized disease. Certainly both physician and patient would profit by the discovery of a diagnostic blood test. It would be simpler and more efficient to take a blood sample from the finger of a suspected patient than to draw pus from the irritated penis or swab the suffering vagina.

Once the diagnosis has been made, the treatment is specific and effective if followed out in disciplined order. Yet, in gonorrhea we meet the problem of penicillin resistance head-on. When penicillin dosage has been increased in the treatment of syphilis, the increase has not been made because of a change in the nature of the spirochete, but rather to ensure that the initial treatment was sufficiently strong to prevent relapse. But the gonococcus has been changing its resistance to drugs from the very start, first, as has been pointed out, to sulfonamides and, more slowly, to penicillin and other antibiotics. The resistance of the gonococcus to sulfonamides developed rapidly. As many as 10 percent were resistant from the start and, in a very short time, resistant strains of gonococci were evident. The sulfonamides also were not always well tolerated, and individual reactions were often quite severe. Naturally, with the introduction of penicillin, in 1944, the medication was regarded as providential. For a decade it appeared that penicillin was again the "miracle" drug, knocking out gonorrhea with apparent success. A friend of mine, to the tune of the Pepsi-Cola jingle, invented a song which ran:

Penicillin that's the stuff
A million units, that's enough
  To cure the syph and the gon-gon, too
Penicillin—that's the dose for you!

However, as time moved on and the resistance to penicillin increased, the words have become less reassuring. Yet, today, penicillin in heavy dosages, in conjunction with a preparation that prolongs its period of activity, is still sometimes the best specific for gonorrhea. In the contemporary study of this disease we must recognize the fact that resistance appears to be particularly prevalent in some parts of the Orient where U.S. armed forces have been stationed. The strains of gonococcus contracted by the men in Korea, Thailand, Vietnam, and elsewhere can be exceptionally strong and resistant to penicillin.

In contrast to syphilis, the treatment of gonorrhea with penicillin seems to be more effective when a quickly absorbed water-soluble solution is given (in a single or repeated dose) instead of one of the slow-acting, slowly absorbed drugs. The idea is to build up the level of penicillin in the blood as high and as fast as possible. Certain other drugs have been used along with penicillin to enhance the effect by slowing excretion of the penicillin through the kidneys. The fact is that in spite of the resistance of the gonococci to penicillin—and the developing resistance to other antibiotics as well—up to now, the effectiveness of either penicillin itself, in sufficient dosage, or one of the newer modified penicillins, or other antibiotics can always be determined simply by testing a culture from the patient, and that drug can be used in treatment. But there is no question as to the fact that there is a contest between the gonococcus and the ingenious chemists. To date, with war, military activity, and the constant moving of bodies around the world, the odds would seem to be mounting on the side of the gonococcus.

The characteristics of gonorrhea make it a pretty unlikely candidate for a good vaccine at this writing. The gonococcus has all of the complexity and more of bacteria as a class. It is only rarely transported into the blood in the course of the disease, and then only in the advanced stages. The natural disease leaves no recognizable immunity, nor does the lack of natural immunity seem to be related to another type variation. Possibly the lack of natural immunity is associated with the characteristic pattern of growth of gonococci *inside* phagocytic cells which, instead of destroying them as would ordinarily be expected, provide nests for them and help to transport them around.

Naturally the possibility of a vaccine for gonorrhea is constantly being explored.* The same attempts at discovering a blood test for gonorrhea also aim, as a by-product, at producing an immunizing agent. There have been reasonably successful efforts to maintain a fully virulent culture, and an experiment has been conducted that produced experimental gonorrhea in chimpanzees, a disease that previously afflicted no other animal except man himself.

However, we must face up to the fact that gonorrhea is raging through the United States at a record rate according to recent statistics of the American Social Health Association. During the fiscal year 1972, the incidence of gonorrhea was the highest it has been in fifty-three years—since the U.S. Public Health Service began to keep records on venereal disease in 1919. It is estimated that there were at least 2,500,000 new cases of gonorrhea in 1972. Even with these figures we must be cognizant of the fact that many cases of gonorrhea are not detected and that many are treated and not reported, so that the actual incidence of the disease cannot be known. Overall, gonorrhea continues to be uncontrolled in most areas. There is, however, some evidence of a reduction of the reservoir of asymptomatic female gonorrhea

*At the time of this writing a simple blood test for gonorrhea is being investigated and used experimentally in some of the metropolitan areas. The most recent reports have been encouraging.

through screening programs and contact investigation. This trend may offer some hope for its eventual control, but the picture is not very bright.

The reader must know that gonorrhea is an annoying and disabling disease, and may become threatening and dangerous. A patient suspecting the presence of gonorrhea should place himself under the charge of a licensed physician immediately and follow the doctor's instructions *exactly.* At no time should the gonorrheal patient risk his or her health on the basis of the casual advice passed out freely by the well-meaning but uninstructed. One should never rely upon drugstore medication unless it is prescribed by a physician, and preferably by the patient's own physician.

The discharge is always contagious. When infected or suspecting infection the patient should wash his hands carefully with soap and water. Dressings, cotton, etc., should be wrapped in paper and burned or destroyed in an antiseptic container. Soiled linens and towels should not be left around for others to use, although it is with a dubious eye that a physician accepts such a source of contact as being legitimate. Hands should be kept away from the eyes because of the natural affinity of the gonococcus for damp mucous membranes. Any eye irritation should be checked immediately.

One of the most important conditions the gonorrheal patient has to accept is that he must avoid any sexual contact until he is cured. Sexual contacts are liable to carry a fresh infection, and sexual excitement is dangerous to the patient and tends to seat the disease more deeply, making it harder to cure. Failure to abstain from sexual contact during the period of treatment is one of the reasons that many cases of gonorrhea become chronic.

While gonorrhea, in general, is not threatening to life, it can cause blindness, crippling arthritis, sterility, and other physical aberrations. It is probably three to four times as prevalent as syphilis, and its toll in suffering and invalidism is enormous, while the money loss and physical disabilities are staggering. For the most part, the age group infected is younger than that of syphilis, although today the presence of both diseases in the same person is not uncommon. An acquaintance who is a gynecologist with a practice consisting of exceptionally promiscuous patients, told me he jokingly greeted a new patient with a jocular: "Anybody going for VD today? . . . Two for the price of one." His mock levity is countermanded by his actual seriousness, and the remark is meant to alleviate the surprise of the patient in whom he has discovered gonorrhea when he insists on a test for syphilis.

Reinfection with gonorrhea occurs with great frequency and regularity. Among homosexuals, gonorrhea has been steadily on the incline. The most common form, other than urethral gonorrhea, is anorectal. As in women, the incubation period can be longer and the original infection may not disturb the infected person immediately, so that when the condition is seen by a physician, the disease has usually already made serious advances.

One of the factors we must take into serious consideration in regard to the increase in the number of people infected with gonorrhea throughout the world is the great danger recently noted of a marked increase in gonorrheal infection of the eyes of newborn babies. This tragic disease, which is technically called gonorrheal conjunctivitis or ophthalmia neonatorum, may swiftly result in blindness in an infant born to a mother who has gonorrhea. This gonorrheal conjunctivitis in a baby results from contamination of the child's eyes during birth. As we know, the bacteria that cause gonorrhea thrive only in certain tissues of the human body and can be transmitted only by direct contact with the discharge from an infected surface, such as the male urethra or female vagina. The epithelium of the eye of a baby that is being born is conducive to the growth of the gonorrheal organism. Thus the infected mother transmits the disease to the baby as it journeys through the birth canal.

Signs of the eye infection generally do not appear until

forty-eight hours have elapsed after birth. Usually both eyes become swollen although, occasionally, only one eye is involved. If treatment is not given, the cornea ulcerates and the infection spreads inside the eyeball, quickly causing blindness. In fact, without treatment, over 90 percent of the babies infected with gonorrheal conjunctivitis will lose their vision. Unfortunately, at a period when there is a constant increase in world evidence of the spread of gonorrhea, and a concomitant incidence of gonorrheal conjunctivitis, there has been a great deal of confusion regarding the proper methods of diagnosis and treatment that accompanied growing medical attention to the problem. Again, the reasons underlying the present controversy concerning the management of gonorrheal conjunctivitis is being revealed by studying the history of medical knowledge about this condition.

The relationship between genital disease in the mother and ocular infection in the infant was noted on separate occasions by three different doctors in the eighteenth century; Quellmalz in 1750, Goetz in 1791, and Gibson in 1808, all of whom observed a connection between a malady then known as "babies' sore eyes" and the presence of a vaginal discharge in the mother. At this time, in accordance with prevalent theories as to the origin of diseases, doctors explained to mothers with babies who had lost their eyesight at birth that it was due to vague atmospheric conditions, particularly sudden chilling, which also was the prevalent theory about the origin of the common cold. But in the latter part of the nineteenth century, with the emerging knowledge of the bacterial etiology of disease, intensive studies were made in the relationship of the baby's eyes to the mother's vaginal discharge. When Neisser isolated the gonococcus in 1879, the link was forged. Despite this discovery, no adequate treatment for genital infections was available. Consequently, much attention was directed toward preventing the ocular infection from occurring in the first place.

In 1881, Karl Credé, director of an obstetrical hospital in Leipzig, recommended the use of a 2 percent solution of silver nitrate to be dropped into the eyes of all newborn babies in order to kill the incipient germs and "provide prophylaxis against the development of the full-blown disease."

It was Lucien Howe at Harvard who campaigned for passage of legislation to make instillation of silver nitrate into the eyes of newborn infants compulsory. As a result, by 1926 twenty states in the United States had passed legislation making the Credé treatment mandatory; the incidence of gonorrheal conjunctivitis decreased to such an extent that whereas in 1908 gonorrheal conjunctivitis was responsible for 28 percent of the blindness among new entrants into schools for the blind, by 1950 the percentage had dropped to only 1 percent.

The silver-nitrate method of prophylaxis became a standard procedure in both America and in Europe, the only change being that the dosage in Credé's formula was diminished from 2 to 1 percent. This was done because the original formula was inherently a substance that often caused chemical conjunctivitis, and cases of gonorrheal conjunctivitis were mistakenly reported despite the prophylaxis. In addition, the harm caused by the occasional erroneous use of the stronger solution led a number of physicians to question the value of silver nitrate.

Concurrently, penicillin was noted not only to be effective in treatment of established cases of gonorrheal conjunctivitis, but to have a prophylactic value as well when administered in local drops or ointments. Since the application of penicillin topically was easy, nonpainful, and nonirritating, it received widespread acceptance. In the United States today, some sort of prophylaxis is legally required in every state, but the regulations vary widely, some using penicillin ointment, others using silver nitrate, and still others using intramuscular penicillin. In many European countries (notably in England) the compulsory use of some form of prophylaxis in the eyes of newborn infants has been abandoned.

The truth is that gonorrheal conjunctivitis is a *preventable* disease. Unfortunately, no reliable screening test exists, such as the serologic blood test which is available for syphilis; and, therefore, a large number of female patients remain in whom it is difficult to detect the presence of gonorrhea. In light of the recent increase of this infection in the adult population, the risk of blindness caused by the presence of gonorrhea in the mother has also increased. To prevent the tragic consequences of this form of VD, the expectant mother should not rely upon antibiotics to eliminate her infection; she should be aware that she could be the victim of a new infection just before the birth of her baby, and of the risk that the infant might be born with gonorrheal conjunctivitis. She should insist upon proper preventative prophylaxis regardless of existing or nonexisting laws. The maintenance of control of gonorrheal conjunctivitis, particularly with the epidemic proportions of gonorrhea today, is one of the challenges of modern medicine, concentrating as it does on prevention rather than cure, an ounce being worth more than a pound in this instance.

In past years, one of the great tragedies of gonorrhea was the effect of the disease upon marriage, since a woman may harbor the disease for a greater length of time and might only be infectious at certain periods. She may harbor the germs and pass them on to infect another with the disease and still show no evidence of ever having had gonorrhea. Many cases have been reported where both husband and wife are infected, neither one quite cured at the same time, and spreading the infection back and forth in Ping-Pong fashion. The effect of gonorrhea upon the child-bearing role of the wife and mother cannot be overstated nor too dramatically highlighted.

As with syphilis, the control of gonorrhea revolves, for the time being, around whether the patient reveals the source of contact and the possible tranference since infection. Again, it is a tedious, thankless job . . . a job of pleading, cajoling, and even threatening and, at best, the results are somewhat nebulous. Again we are involved in emotions, in the delicate structure of personal relationships of deceit and revenge. With proper knowledge, we might shift the responsibility to the individual affected with VD; but our understanding of human frailty and people's tendency to "pass the buck" and dismiss the unpleasant, leads us to relegate the hope for such control to the brimming basket of failure.

In our practices and in our professional intercommunications, we physicians realize that when VD is caught in time, and treated properly, it can be controlled—if the patient will cooperate and be true to himself as well as to others. He must be ready to assume his portion of the blame and to follow through in informing others involved regardless of how painful the situation or how damaging to his or her personal relationship. VD is not a plaything; it is a deathtrap for man's most creative and procreative force.

4

VENEREAL DISEASE IN PREGNANCY: THE UNBORN INNOCENTS

In view of the fact that venereal disease is primarily a disease of the young, and that youth is the period of pregnancy, it seems pertinent that the effects of venereal disease upon expectant parents should be covered in detail.

Not only are the young more inclined to be romantic in heart, they are usually the least informed age group in regard to the contraction of venereal disease or the really serious consequences attending it. Like Scarlett O'Hara, most young people tend to put aside any unpleasant responsibilities with a simple "I'll think about it tomorrow" attitude.

Despite the major efforts to eradicate the gonococcus from our society, efforts made through enlightened epidemiological control, modern diagnostic methods, and the use of new antibiotics, the gonococcus, like the rat, continues to flourish. It has been said by Dr Thorstein Güthe of the World Health Organization that no method has yet been found of "catching up with this heelless Achilles." One of the problems in controlling the disease is the general attitude among the laity—and especially among the young—of indifference towards gonorrhea. Too many young people think of gonorrhea as a trifling disease that can be cured by a visit to a drugstore or the use of a remedy recommended by a compeer. In Public Health Centers, the attempts at control have resulted in so many insurmountable problems that any hope often goes aglimmering. Years ago physicians handled *all* cases of urethritis, but today the vast majority are *resistant* cases, that come to him because self-treatment has failed. The short incubation period makes it possible for the disease to spread rapidly, and, as noted previously, the difficulty of diagnosis in the female presents a formidable problem. Gonorrhea remains one of the number-one enemies of the institution of marriage. In the male if the disease is not checked in time, sterility results, and in the female, not only does the disease cause sterility, but it can produce chronic ill-health which can mar the sexual happiness of married life.

Let me state right from the start that unless there are skin manifestations to indicate the presence of an eruptive venereal disease, VD in pregnancy and in parenthood belongs in the office of the gynecologist-obstetrician for the female, and in the office of the urologist for the male, rather than in the office of the syphilologist. If there is a skin eruption that might lead the boy or girl to a syphilologist, he would naturally refer them to the proper specialists for prenatal and postnatal care of the parents and of the newborn infant.

We have illustrated that chronic pelvic inflammatory ailment in women and blindness in infants born of women infected with gonorrhea are two of the serious consequences of this disease if allowed to go unchecked. Certainly any young girl who is pregnant should be constantly examined for the presence of gonorrhea. Unfortunately, many young mothers do not procure medical care until the last month of pregnancy, and sometimes not until the hour of delivery.

Like a thief in the night who, under cover of darkness, follows his victim until he is vulnerable and unprotected and then pounces, syphilis, the arch destroyer of fetal life, hides behind the mother's relative immunity until the protecting early months of pregnancy are passed, and then, when the barriers against its invasion are removed, invades the fetal membranes and destroys its innocent victim, the unborn child.

The response of the organism of infection in the gravid woman is even less typical than in the nonpregnant woman. Primary lesions are rarely observed and, when they do occur, may be multiple and often small and quite atypical. Occasionally, however, the opposite is true, and because of the increased vascularity of the parts, the chancre is larger, is more indurated, and lasts much longer than that of the nonpregnant woman. Secondary manifestations are mild unless they are situated on the genitalia where they are larger and more numerous, and where they more frequently become ulcerated. In the majority of cases of syphilitic pregnant women, the disease is latent or its symptoms are so mild that, unless serological studies are made, the prospective mother is unaware of infection until a miscarriage or premature stillbirth directs attention to the underlying cause. This consistent mildness or total absence of symptoms justifies the belief that women, and especially pregnant women, possess some protective agent that tends to check the ravages of syphilis. Accordingly women, especially those who have been pregnant after infection, should be less likely to develop serious late manifestations of syphilis. It is true that both cardiovascular and neurosyphilis are over twice as common in male syphilitics as in female syphilitics.

The response of the products of conception to infection is as severe as that of the maternal organism is slight. Protected as it is in the early months, the fetus continues to develop normally until about the middle of the pregnancy when it is apparently overwhelmed by the invading host of spirochetes that pass through the altered placental barrier Unless the spirochetes have been weakened by long contact with the mother's protecting mechanism, this general invasion of the helpless fetus soon leads to its destruction. In the case of women who have recently been infected, death and expulsion of the fetus commonly occur in the fifth and sixth months; latent cases carry their pregnancies longer, but, ultimately, the disease manifests itself in either premature and full-term stillbirths or in the birth of living syphilitic infants. The results should point to the fact that although pregnancy may help the mother's syphilis, that same syphilis will almost always destroy her unborn child.

Since the usual evidences of infection are mild or masked in most women, and since the disease tends to be latent during pregnancy, the only practical way of recognizing syphilis in pregnancy is by the use of blood tests. If these tests are not given routinely, the majority of cases will go unsuspected until a late abortion, a premature stillbirth, or the birth of a syphilitic infant will demonstrate the tragic consequences of neglect and lack of prenatal care which occurs so often among the young and the impoverished.

When we consider that it is now estimated that 10 percent of the population between the ages of fifteen and twenty-four years (estimate by the public health officials of California in 1972) are infected with either syphilis or gonorrhea or both, we must look towards tomorrow's children. As taxpayers and citizens we must face the responsibility involved in the facts. Many of our child-bearing females are in the indigent or near-indigent groups. During pregnancy they get little or no prenatal care, and since they often live in a physical and social environment in which syphilis is an ever-present risk, they, unfortunately, are vulnerable to producing syphilitic babies who are either born dead or damaged. So despite the fact that, intellectually and medically, VD in pregnancy is a "controlled" situation, in reality it is not.

Congenital Syphilis

In the past decade, the increase in congenital syphilis has paralleled the incidence in the rise of reported syphilis among adults. In the Los Angeles County-University of Southern

California Medical Center it is estimated that there are twice as many cases of congenital syphilis as were seen five years earlier. According to hospital authorities, syphilis has been the transplacental infection most often encountered in the nurseries in the last four years. In descending order are rubella, herpes virus hominus, and cytomegalic inclusion disease. The typical bone lesions seen in congenital syphilis are the easiest aid to early diagnosis; rhinitis and maculopapular rash follow in due order. But many infants who are ill from birth present none of the specific signs and symptoms associated with transplancental infections of various kinds. Consequently, clinical diagnosis is most difficult in early cases and, in congenital syphilis, prompt and early recognition is most important because effective treatment is available. Recently, at the Los Angeles County-USC Medical Center six cases of congenital syphilis in newborns were studied; in four, the condition was diagnosed shortly after birth. The two remaining patients were discharged asymptomatic from the nursery and returned with symptoms when two or three months of age. Because these cases are rather typical of the general problem of the diagnosis of the disease, the treatment and the lack of follow-up, I present them so that the reader can gain some perception of the danger of the presence of venereal disease in the pregnant mother and the effect upon the newborn infant.

Case 1: A child was born to a woman whose pregnancy was uneventful with the exception of a mild episode of flulike illness with rash lasting fifteen days during the last month of pregnancy. A Venereal Disease Research Laboratory (VDRL) test for syphilis on blood drawn in the first trimester of pregnancy was positive, but the mother was lost to public health check-up. At birth the infant was depressed, and in the nursery she had rapid respirations. The extremities were edematous and the face puffy. Tests were taken on the cord blood and were positive. The infant was given fluids intravenously and penicillin and digitalis parenterally. On the second day a rash appeared. Radiographs showed the typical lesions of congenital syphilis in the long bones. The child remained critically ill for six days and then gradually improved and was dismissed from the nursery in good condition in three weeks. When last seen at two months no neurological nor physical abnormality was present. The mother returned to Mexico and the infant was lost to further follow-up.

Case 2: A girl born to a mother who had one prenatal clinic visit and the VDRL test drawn at that time was negative. At birth, the baby was wrinkled and had poor muscle tone. On the fifth day she developed respiratory difficulties and an X-ray of the long bones showed congenital syphilis. Penicillin therapy was administered and the infant left the clinic at the end of two weeks of therapy. When last seen at three months, there was evident healing of the lesions in the long bones. Follow-up discontinued.

Case 3: A premature girl baby born to a young woman who had no prenatal care and was admitted to the hospital in active labor. The infant had peeling skin and generalized poor muscle tone. Radiographs showed congenital syphilis. The child was treated with penicillin and dismissed at the end of two weeks. When last seen at the age of three months she was alert, active, and growing well although her right leg was shorter than the left and had limited movement. Case lost from that date.

Case 4: A premature baby born to a young woman with no prenatal care who was admitted to the hospital with vaginal bleeding and in active labor. At delivery, the infant was severely depressed, limp, and gasping. The lungs were filled with mucus and the abdomen distended. Pneumonia set in and despite intravenous fluids and penicillin treatment the infant died after five hours of life. The post-mortem showed congenital syphilis rampant throughout the entire body.

Case 5: A baby girl born of a mother who had no prenatal care. Pregnancy was normal and delivery uncomplicated. Baby was normal at birth and discharged before positive results of tests for syphilis on the mother's blood were reported. Infant was lost to follow-up, but at two and a half months the infant was returned to the out-patient department with a rash on the palms and a complaint of tenderness and depressed movement of the left leg. Long-bone radiographs showed multiple destructive bone lesions consistent with congenital syphilis. The infant was admitted to the hospital and given penicillin treatment and released at the end of two weeks in good condition. One month later she was improving with healing of lesions; no further follow-up.

Case 6: A boy born to a woman who came from Mexico eight months before delivery having received no prenatal care. Pregnancy and delivery were uncomplicated. The infant was normal at birth and discharged before the mother's serologic tests were reported positive for syphilis. The infant was referred for evaluation to the hospital clinic at two weeks of age. He was alert, active, and well nourished. Radiographs of the long bones were normal. Results of VDRL tests were normal. He was discharged from the clinic at one month without treatment.

At two and a half months he was admitted to the hospital with redness and limitation of movement of the right upper arm. On admission, he appeared alert and well nourished. Radiographs of the long bones showed multiple destructive lesions consistent with congenital syphilis. VDRL tests were positive. After treatment with parenteral penicillin for two weeks the baby was discharged in good condition. When last seen at four and a half months he was alert, active, and developing normally.

The cases have been reported here to illustrate the importance of syphilitic examinations of the mother during prenatal care and, when that is absent, the importance of early diagnosis in the newborn infant with continuing pediatric treatment. As we can see, the response to the treatment was excellent in all cases except for the one baby that expired.

What of those infants who are born congenital syphilitics? "A little, wrinkled, pot-bellied old man with a cold in his head," to quote the famous description by P. Diday, who wrote a very clear and concise monograph upon the subject of congenital syphilis in 1888. In addition to his description, there are other symptoms that were observed. The snuffles mentioned above are highly characteristic; the skin of the typical congenital syphilitic is dry and leathery; his temporal arteries are as hard and tortuous as those of an old man of eighty years who is dying of arteriosclerosis; his entire body is covered with eruptions that are raw and oozing; there are mucus patches in the mouth and on the gums and many shallow ulcerations and warty growths about the genitals and the organs of excretion. In nearly all of these lesions *Treponema pallidum* can be discovered by the use of the darkfield illuminator. (Fortunately, unlike other forms of disease, persons with congenital syphilis show a lasting immunity against redevelopment of any other stages of the disease.)

The congenital syphilitic has always furnished the most bizarre examples of diseases that attack mankind. If these unfortunates were able to reach adolescence and maturity and, perchance, old age, many of them would have developed manifestations that set them apart from other persons. These manifestations, called the stigmata of syphilis, are almost totally of bone and eye, central nervous system and skin involvement. For many years it was not known that there is an early and late stage of latency in the congenital as well as in the acquired type of syphilis, and that the disease may be latent in the congenital type for as long as thirty-five to fifty years before overt signs of the disease appear, and some may never show any indication of their disease. But, ordinarily, the spirochete, in attacking the embryo so interferes with the developments of these parts that the infants show manifestations when they are born or soon thereafter.

Of all the manifestations the worst involvement in the congenital syphilitic is that of the central nervous system. Optic atrophy is not unknown, and brain syphilis, taboparesis, and juvenile paresis are commonplace. It is believed that 25 percent of all congenital syphilitics have some type of nervous-system involvement, as shown by examination of the spinal fluid of these children.

There seems to be a neurotropic strain of the *Treponema pallidum.* Sometimes the iris of the eye in taboparetics degenerates until the body of that organ becomes a thin black line. The taroparetic pupil reacts neither to light nor accommodation. The juvenile paretic and the taboparetic nearly always die young in spite of all treatment including malarial fever, penicillin, or any other kind of modern therapy. If these victims live long enough, it is to exist only as vegetables, "sans teeth, sans eyes, sans taste, sans everything" (*As You Like It,* Shakespeare).

The serologic findings may become entirely negative and if, by chance, they are admitted to a mental hospital in later years, the medical staff may be hard put to make a diagnosis of paresis or taboparesis because all tests are negative. A study of juvenile paretics was made by William Menninger, Udo J. Wile, and Charles C. Dennie. The conclusions were all the same–*prognosis negative.* Except for the humanitarian aspect, it is almost useless to treat such cases.

It has taken a little over four centuries of the combined efforts of physicians, biologists, chemists, physicists, and neuropsychiatrists to put together the jigsaw puzzle of the syphilitic disease into one solid picture. In order to do this they had to discover the almost perfect cure, penicillin. Syphilitic pregnant mothers, properly treated at the proper time with penicillin, deliver healthy babies 98 percent of the time. And, there is a place for the congenital syphilitics and their children, under proper management. It is to obtain such goals that we need public education about syphilis and prompt treatment. There cannot be too vigorous a pursuit of both goals by doctors and public alike. Until such a date, the story will remain one of tragedy for the uninformed and untreated mother and for her innocently mutilated, unborn child.

5

THE "SOCIAL DISEASES"

In its basic definition, the word "social" means "marked by pleasant companionship with one's friends"; or "relating to human society, the interaction of the group and its members, and the welfare of those members."

In the terminology of syphilis and gonorrhea as "social" diseases, we assume the broad aspect of the effect of these contagious diseases, not only upon the individual as a patient, but upon the individual as a part of the society in which he lives. We accept the fact that VD exists, that VD can be cured and controlled as a medical problem, but that, to date, the specific—penicillin—has failed to eradicate the problem and that the diseases are in our midst in what is regarded as epidemic incidence. With the tools we possess, what to do?

One social worker whom I consulted suggested that VD could only be curtailed by a change in the free-wheeling sexual behavior of people. Another advocated better sex education for the young, which would give them an increased understanding of the diseases and their effects upon society.

Films, the press, cosmetic firms, dress designers have all concentrated exaggeratedly on sexual attraction. One of the airlines has had a very successful advertising campaign in which attractive young girls urge the onlooker "to come on and fly me," my name is Mary, Jane, or Helen—with the subtle sexual innuendo left in the air and in the viewer's imagination. How can the suggestion of a change in sexual behavior patterns stand up to the constant barrage of the importance of an unreal world of sexual attraction? It is resolved intellectually by the fact that for every person impelled to promiscuity (promiscuity defined as frequent and indiscriminate choice of sexual partners) by these external influences, there can be found an individual who has resisted them; the individual character and personality, the psychological make-up, being the determining factor.

It was Dr. Thomas Parran who suggested many years ago that VD be isolated from its social category and be regarded strictly as a problem of disease—a contagious and dangerous disease. Most doctors will agree with Dr. Parran that VD should be sequestered from its social implications, and that it should be treated as unembellished disease. It is only in this manner that we will ever obtain any degree of control with the tools with which we have to work. But we are fighting a battle of the centuries, of moralisms and pietisms versus reality and reason.

VD developed out of the circumstances of man's progress on earth; and from the fragmentary historical evidence of its scope in early times, it reached a frightening vertex during the Renaissance, and continued on a set course until recent times, when again it has soared to an even more marked and exaggerated degree. Today, it is brought together in apocalyptic fashion as just another one of the great problems confronting our society. Poverty, sloth, ignorance, lack of proper medical facilities: All contribute to the spread of VD. If we could eradicate all the elements I have just mentioned, we could also palliate the emotional insecurity which is the underlying basis for man's sexual promiscuity. But to change the nature of man is of an order of greater magnitude than the eradication of VD, and a quite unachievable Utopian dream.

That VD is spread by sexual contact means that its incidence is naturally increased as sexual intercourse in the population increases and, with promiscuity an essential factor in the process, we must accept the fact that VD is going to accelerate within a sexually promiscuous society. Obviously there is more VD amongst the poor than among the rich—primarily because the rich are usually more enlightened and have medical facilities more easily available to them. But I can assure you there is no lack of venereal disease at any level of society. Perhaps it is more shocking if one contracts VD from a clean-cut, intelligent member of society than from an uninformed, sexually promiscuous individual, but it happens with unfailing regularity.

What is needed is neither sociological nor moralistic, but technological. *Syphilis needs a vaccine and gonorrhea needs a simple diagnostic test in addition.* Since at this writing neither exists, we must get back to the social factors in the VD problem: lack of sex education, prostitution and homosexuality, and an answer as to why people fail to go for medical treatment, or if they do go, cease the treatment before the cure is affected, and why they refuse to reveal the sexual contacts to whom they have transferred the disease.

What is meant by sex education?

Sex education begins with an honest examination of anatomy, physiology, embryology, and genetics. It cannot begin too young in response to the natural curiosity of the child. To argue whether it should be taught in the home or in the school is academic, the essential point being that it should be taught in the natural course of events as part of the processes of life. All the ramifications of the sexual process are part of life, and are natural and clean and beautiful; only when crippled by disease are these aspects destroyed. The understanding and simple hygienic care of the genitals is the first step towards introducing VD without lies or hypocriscy. The importance of the care of the female organs as receptacles of childbearing, if taught early enough, would help many a young girl endure the trials of puberty, and would help her lay a foundation for a healthy attitude towards love and sex that would preclude sexual promiscuity. That love tends to create love is not merely an aphorism of the poet.

In the course of the child's sex education such problems as homosexuality, pregnancy, abortion, and VD should be treated with honesty. I believe the adult, in teaching sex education, should assume a somewhat passive role, answering but not imposing. Certainly no set, unbreakable rules should be laid down to a child or an adolescent by an adult. Guidance rather than dogmatic teaching would be the ideal course; the parent, or the adult, should be sufficiently informed and unbiased to answer the questions to the satisfaction of the inquirer. To deny the existence of homosexuality to a growing child is as dangerous as to deny the possibility of pregnancy to a young girl who has commenced menstruating. But above all, in all forms of sex education, the beauty of the sex life of a man and woman, unimpaired by ignorance and old-hat puritanical mores cannot be overly stressed.

Much effort is expended to achieve the "body beautiful"; the young person should know that the body beautiful is the body devoid of disease. I have been asked by many people what I would recommend in the prevention of VD and I find myself always replying with the old adage: "A little soap and water never hurt anyone!" The therapeutic value of learning to clean the genitals properly in childhood is amazing. Add this to the knowledge that in the erotic areas, the aroused germs of Venus will live and thrive unless washed away by the elementary means of using soap and water.

At first glance, it may seem that bringing prostitution into a manuscript written in 1973 is a bit of an anachronism. Yet, in this era of sexual freedom on a scale larger than ever previously condoned, the prosperity enjoyed by this institution is confirmed by statistics. Why? we ask automatically, why prostitution when sex is available for free? The answer is twofold: First, a person may want to become a prostitute today not only because of the guilt and self-destructive impulses described by Freud, but because of the money involved (and, perhaps, because contemporary society has cast a certain glamor on the job of call girl—Jane Fonda's portrayal in the film *Klute* is an example). The Las Vegas prostitute, by her own admission, earns $50,000 a year. Second, we must consider the role of men who patronize prostitutes because they want no involvement beyond sex and want it limited in time, expense, and concern, as well as those men who become powerful and wealthy as a result of prostitution. These factors serve to perpetuate prostitution.

Prostitution and VD have been bed-partners since the beginning of both; and there is no separating the two, although the prostitute of today will present a reasonable argument that she is less apt to contract a disease than the amateur, and is less apt to be a source of disease because of her wider knowledge of its signs in the male. But the facts do not support her contention. Just as in the past, prostitution and venereal disease are still bedfellows.

Today prostitution has become a legal problem, overlapping into the area of morality. Actually, prostitution, like venereal disease, is a social concern. It has assumed many identities. As an institution, it is not of very ancient, prehistorical vintage; it is thought to have its origins in historical times, when religious rites involved groups of women or men dedicated to a fertility god who practiced prostitution in connection with temple rites. These groups had religious sanction. In the Greek culture, we cannot bypass the hetaeras; in Rome, we witness the day of the concubine; in Japan the geisha. But by this time, prostitution as we know it was already in full bloom, side by side with the courtesan, and concubine, homosexual and heterosexual.

In prewar Europe the sexual education of a young man was often entrusted to an experienced prostitute and there is a romantic aura surrounding the courtesans of the nineteenth century, epitomized by Dumas's *La Dame aux Camélias,* set to music by Verdi in *La Traviata.* In our own time, the movie and the play *Gigi,* based on Colette's delightful story, has brought pleasure to thousands of people. In American history, the role of the prostitute bringing the chi-chi atmosphere and pseudoculture of the famous bordellos of New Orleans to the raw, crude West for the men who went in search of gold, new frontiers, and wealth, and who were only too happy to mate with an itinerant prostitute, is accepted Americana. Our major cities have their legends of prostitutes and houses of prostitution, all of which are part of our national legend. To deny this would be blatant hypocrisy.

The definition of prostitution is: a promiscuous sexual activity which is paid for or which is practiced as a means of earning one's livelihood. In our time, a woman works and lives alone (or, before marriage, with other young women) and has what sexual relations she desires. Today many, if not a majority, of girls have had sexual intercourse before marriage. Most of the girls have not had to resort to prostitution for the need of a "roof overhead." Her resolution to become a prostitute, relying solely on her sex for a livelihood, is usually a combination of psychological factors and sometimes a craving for luxuries which are not allowed for in the average working girl's budget. In a large metropolitan area like Manhattan, prostitution has reached unbelievable proportions. Many attempts have been made, ineffectively, to control both prostitution and venereal disease. Until 1967, the Manhattan division of the Health Department operated a health clinic known as the Criminal Court Clinic where accused prostitutes were examined and treated for VD, and were also offered the alternative of reporting to a private physician or a recognized clinic within forty-eight hours after being freed, in order to control the spread of venereal disease.

In the same year, the long jail term (which had proven ineffective) for streetwalkers was modified to fifteen days in jail and a fine of $250.00. Prostitution was regarded as a social rather than a criminal problem. The result was that New York was besieged with pimps selling whores. New York's midtown area of theaters, restaurants, and hotels became infested with panderers and harlots. It became, and still is, a subject that has been aired by such TV personalities as Johnny Carson and Dick Cavett. The hotels are the main scene of action, with the pimps doing the negotiating and handling of all the legal aspects of the business, leaving the girl free to ply her trade and collect a small amount of the pimp's "take." The result has been "big business" and simultaneously *an alarming increase in the spread of venereal disease.* In addition, the material assets of prostitution seeped into the hinterlands and the amateur prostitute of suburbia became a figure in the American sex scene of the 60s.

Because the increase in VD is international in its epidemic stage, and because we are aware that the moving of human beings from place to place is one means of spreading the diseases and of being unable to check sources and new contacts, we should recognize the fact that prostitution is rampant on an international scale. In Hamburg, Germany, one of the largest port cities of Europe where sailors from all over the world congregate, prostitution is commercially very profitable. In Japan, where brothels were abolished in 1958, prostitution flourishes for the benefit of the visiting sailor and soldier. Saigon, in Vietnam, posed a picture of complete corruption with prostitution accepted as a mode of life, as the number of soldiers exceeded by far the number of women available for sexual pleasure. In Tijuana, Mexican and American import prostitutes ply their trade from morning to night; and in Juarez, another bordertown near the location of the United States armed forces, prostitutes report to clinics for preventative shots of penicillin.

In London, Paris, and the Scandinavian cities, where sexual

freedom among the amateurs is high, admission of venereal disease is also discussed openly, and there is little if any shame attached to getting VD. Medical help is readily solicited, but there is still an incredible amount of ignorance of the medical truths of VD and of the actual role penicillin and antibiotics must play. In these countries, there seems to be a real faith in the curative dominion of the miracle drugs without any substantial knowledge as to the course of the diseases and to the ineffectuality of the drugs in specific instances. The world over, as I have travelled about and encountered different peoples, there seems to be a complacency in the security that venereal disease is something of the past, and that there is no basic problem if one gets his standard dose of penicillin. A voice of caution is like a lost echo in a vast canyon, meaningless sound.

In the world of VD, as we have noted, loose woman is thought of as the culprit, and when we say prostitution, we naturally think of the female of the species. But the sex sale is not restricted to women, and the male prostitute presents just as big a problem as the female. When I first started writing this book and I listed homosexuality as one of the reasons for the current epidemic, a patient of mine, a homosexual, resented my accusation. He questioned whether the increase in venereal disease amonst homosexuals was contributing to the problem. According to the report that was sponsored by the Center of Disease Control of Atlanta, Georgia, and put together by the Seattle-King County Department of Health in the state of Washington in 1970-1971, the proportion of cases of infectious syphilis attributed to homosexual transmission in several cities in Europe and North America has increased from less than 1 percent, prior to 1950, to as many as two-thirds of the cases reported during the past decade. Sixty-five percent of the male patients with infectious syphilis identified homosexual contacts, and the number of cases reported in male homosexuals in 1972 has increased 150 percent over the number reported in the previous year.

The data accumulated by this committee suggests that gonorrhea is more common in male homosexuals than syphilis, but homosexuality is more common among men with syphilis than among men with gonorrhea. Similarly, homosexuality is common among men with granuloma inguinale (GI). The reasons are unclear except that GI is relatively uncommon among females, even among those who are prostitutes, and those who are known to have had sexual contact with men who had GI.

It is interesting to note, that most patients with lymphogranuloma venereum (LVG) have been heterosexual men who contracted the disease outside the United States, usually in the armed services. However, among the men who have contracted the disease within the United States, there have been largely homosexual males hospitalized originally with symptoms of rectal infection.

Until now, data have not been accumulated scientifically on such venereal diseases as chancroid and herpes virus amongst homosexuals.

Obviously, with statistics on venereal diseases among homosexuals available, the question arises, Is homosexuality becoming more common among American males? In 1948, the famous Kinsey Report disclosed that an estimated 37 percent of white adult males in the United States experienced physical homosexual contact at least once during their lives, but only 4 percent were thought to be "predominantly homosexual" at any time. To date, no subsequent studies of any comparable scope have been conducted and sexologists have documented no increase since that time in the proportion of white adult American men who are "predominantly homosexual." Yet the evidence, with the "opening of the closet door," so to speak, and the gradual impact of the "gay liberation" groups, would indicate that the percentage might be higher—or, if not higher, the admission of homosexual identity might be more relaxed than at the time of the Kinsey report, and the statistic would show a higher percentage of admissions. Within the homosexual percentage, there is usually about 29 percent who claim to be bisexual with 3 to 144 sexual contacts with females per year. Thus, a continuum from predominantly homosexual to predominantly heterosexual behavior exists in such men, who may transfer venereal disease from the homosexual to the heterosexual community. Examples are well known to syphilis investigators of microepidemics of syphilis among heterosexuals which have been traced to an initial homosexual male source. (An interview with a male homosexual with syphilis who worked in a "massage parlor" in Los Angeles which catered strictly to the male trade, admitted that a large percentage of his clients were heterosexual men, with wives and families, who admittedly were unfulfilled patrons for the experience of sexual pleasures. The age group of these clients, interestingly, was the middle forties—men experiencing the male change-of-life span.)

The diagnosis of primary syphilis in the male homosexual requires examination of the penis, anal canal, and oral cavity. The low frequency of anal and oral chancres amongst homosexuals indicates that these chancres, like those in women, are infrequently recognized by clinicians and consequently represent a silent reservoir of syphilis among homosexual men. Anal chancres are painless unless accompanied by hemorrhoids or other complications and must be diagnosed by darkfield examination together with appropriate serologic tests. Confirmation of oral chancres are difficult because *Treponema microdentium,* which resembles *Treponema pallidum* is normally present in the mouth.

But, as we have pointed out, the sexual practices—reputedly confined to the homosexual world—are actually common among both homosexuals and the heterosexuals. And this, too, is not unique to this generation of so-called sexual permissiveness—it has been true since the beginning of sexual explorations and pleasures. Possibly the only difference is the availability of communication channels. Unfortunately, those same channels which have revealed the sexual practices of mankind the world over, have failed also to inform the sex voyager of the diseases to be encountered on the sea of sexual adventure.

To understand the position I have taken, one must understand the role of homosexuality in the history of man. The male prostitute, often a passive homosexual, but frequently an aggressive hustler, is not a new phenomenon. He has been in existence for some millenia and is evoked in literature from Aristophanes and Juvenal through Proust and Tennessee Williams. If there is anything new about homosexuality, it is merely its current acceptance and the evidences of it seen about us which, in intervening generations, was restricted to limited areas and identified by the expression "closet queen." It must also be recognized that homosexuals cannot be identified positively by either sex, race, age, dress, mannerism, or marital status.

To investigate this study beyond my own practice, I visited the VD Clinic sponsored by the Gay Liberation movement in Los Angeles. The incidence of venereal disease among the gay set was extremely high, and the visitors to the clinic included many homosexuals who went to the clinic instead of visiting their own doctors because, despite the numbers of patients, there is a certain anonymity in a clinic, and a fraternal experience, instead of an isolated one.

In the analysis of VD among homosexuals, the male homosexual is more prone to be the recipient of VD than the female homosexual, for Lesbians tend—as one friend of mine has often said—"to imitate middle-class men" and set up an imitative marital relationship without legal sanction, remaining reasonably faithful sexually to one partner at a time, whereas the male homosexual is generally more promiscuous. In addition, male homosexuality frequently involves pederasty, so that the lesions and symptoms in the passive member are usually found in the anorectal area, where—especially in the case of syphilis—they present the same diagnostic difficulties that one finds in syphilis of the vagina in females.

The original chancre is painless and often not observed, so that, frequently, until the patient is in the second or third stage, or until some other symptom occurs, the patient is ignorant of his disease and is transmitting it with all the frequency his libido permits. In the case of gonorrhea, the male homosexual may suffer pains in the rectum similar to those endured by the female in the vagina. His attention is then drawn to his condition; but, very often, unless his partner suffers urethral pain, the patient with gonorrhea in the rectum might ignore the condition, just as a woman might, until it has penetrated into deeper tissues, or other complications arise.

Certainly, if there is more VD amongst homosexuals today, it can be attributed to the sliding rule of numbers; i.e., more men are openly admitting to having committed acts of homosexuality than previously, and the practicing homosexual feels freer to express himself sexually. Any study of homosexuality recognizes that the "quest" and the "conquest" are part of the sexual drive. In addition, the youth appeal in which sex is at its peak, is one of the factors that compose the identity of the homosexual. To fortify one's feeling of sexual attraction and desirability, sexual episodes are essential; consequently, promiscuity is part and parcel of the average homosexual personality.

While most homosexual prostitution is carried on by street and bar solicitation, there is a modern version of the bordello which exists for males as well as females—the "massage parlor" and the "baths." These once respected places of recuperation from overindulgence in drink or from actual physical fatigue have fallen into disrepute in the past decade or so, and today are usually places of sexual assignation. The customer feels a certain safety and anonymity within the steambath walls, for the place is usually police protected. Most prostitutes working in these locations are inspected for venereal disease regularly and, if afflicted, are suspended from activity. But again, alas, the chances of contracting VD considering the large number of customers encountered, gives VD an edge in the odds. The income of male and female prostitutes working in massage parlors may vary from $100 to $500 per day. It is difficult, under the stress of economic pressure, to moralize or to prescribe a change in sexual behavior to a good working whore, male or female.

The third part of the study of the social diseases as related to their social aspect ("social" defined as the interaction of the members of a group working for the general welfare) are persistent questions that beset the doctor. Why does the infected person fail to come for medical help? Why, if they do, do they fail to undergo the complete treatment? Why will they not willingly give the names of the contacts they have encountered? *Why?*

Actually, if I could answer the *why*, I might qualify not only as a medical syphilologist, but as a competent practitioner of psychiatry as well, for the question involves the behavior patterns of past generations and the thoughts deeply rooted in the subconscious of men and women of today—thoughts associating sex with sin, and sin with punishment.

Despite the fact that we doctors, for the most part, try to isolate VD simply as a disease comparable to any other contagious disease such as tuberculosis, we are fighting a losing battle with the attitude of the patient. The presence of VD in the patient is self-revelatory; it is a condition in which the patient knows that the doctor is aware of the conditions under which he or she contracted the disease, i.e., through sexual cohabitation. If the patient could accept the fact that the doctor is not a moral censor and that he has no interest in the details of the sexual encounter that produced the disease—other than to be certain that the other party is cautioned to seek medical help—much of the control of VD could be accomplished. But, very often, the doctor finds himself administering a single-dose treatment against his better medical judgment because he is fully aware that he will never again see the patient, and that further treatment will either be neglected or sought elsewhere, where the patient is still an unknown.

Obviously the answer lies in the fact that there is still a certain element of shame identified with VD. Shame is defined as a sense of guilt, and guilt carries with it a fear of punishment. Obviously, no doctor is going to punish his patient for having VD, but there is no way except through individual and highly personal doctor-patient relationships that this sort of understanding can occur.

In the case of VD, the doctor's office becomes not unlike the confessional booth, and the doctor is obliged to assume a role which is not his. Regardless of the conditions under which the patient was infected—whether sordid, exotic, or commonplace—the doctor's only concern is the condition of the disease and the patient. When did it occur? How far has it progressed? What contacts has the patient had since the one when he was infected? All the pertinent facts are merely "portion of the case history" devised to help the doctor help the patient. It is not probing for curiosity's sake, nor is it moral censure. Because of lack of education, the patient does not understand that the shot of penicillin is not going to be the cure-all, the ultimate panacea. Cooperation and communication between the doctor and the patient are essential, and if the right attitude is established, the patient can be definitively cured. Also, through frank talks with the doctor, some rapport might emerge that would enable the doctor to discuss the patient's overall sexual status, and lead to the recommendation of proper care and prevention after the disease is under control.

Many people maintain that sick people would seek help if only they knew they were sick. Perhaps so; but the fears associated with VD are of such proportions that a doctor such as myself may see many people enter the office gingerly with a skin eruption and not knowing what their sickness is, yet somehow, automatically associating skin eruptions with VD as they tensely await the diagnosis. I am convinced that with all of our sexual emancipation, there is still a reluctance on the part of human beings to discuss VD openly.

Of course, there is the exception to the rule, as in the patient who boasts of VD as he or she boasts of sexual conquests, but such characters are not as common as we are led to believe. Most patients suspecting VD are *scared*—and reassurance does not come easily. In the role of the syphilologist who diagnoses VD usually because of the presence of some skin eruption, the keeping of case histories is a most formidible task, because the recognition and diagnosis very often strain the doctor-patient relationship. It is tragic that with all of the emphasis upon sex today, a guide cannot be provided as to the chances of contracting VD and the need for immediate and proper medical diagnosis and care. Force will not control VD, nor will police regulations control promiscuity, nor punishment avail to prevent infection.

To follow simple rules of genital cleanliness is essential, and the knowledge that, today, in the book of odds, if one plays freely at the sex game, a physician should be available in whom one can confide, and a periodical physical examination is of the utmost importance.

No one is invulnerable.

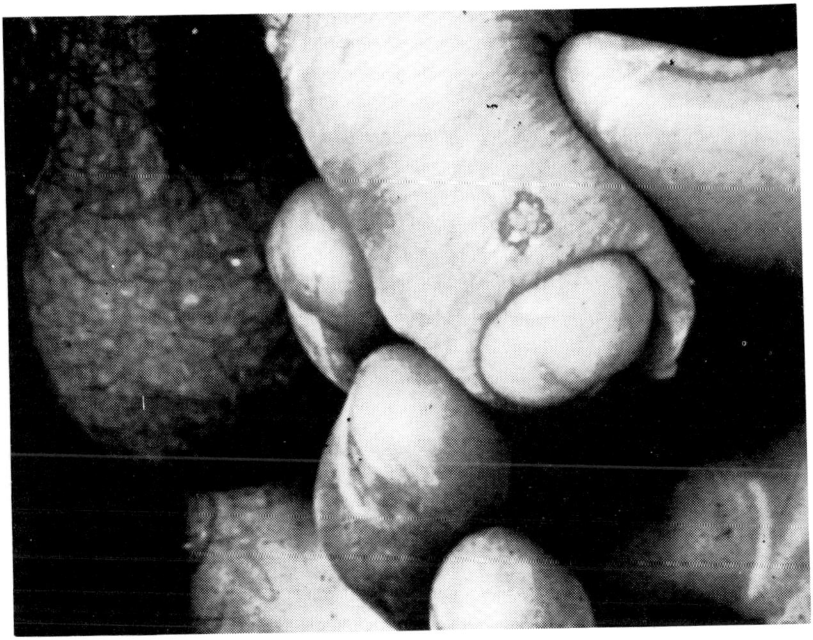

1. Primary syphilis. Chancre on the foreskin.

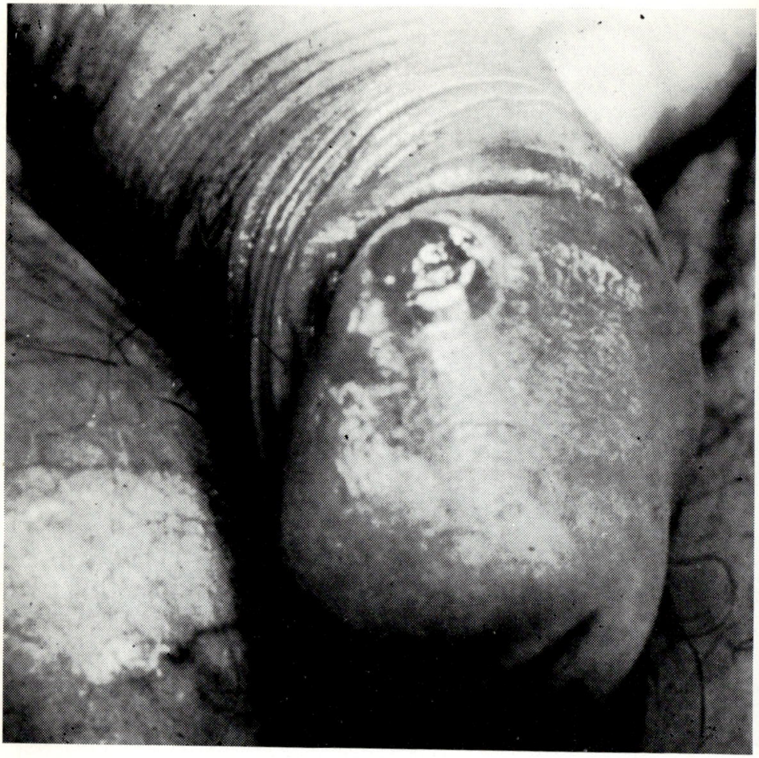

2. *Primary syphilis. Chancre on the glans penis.*

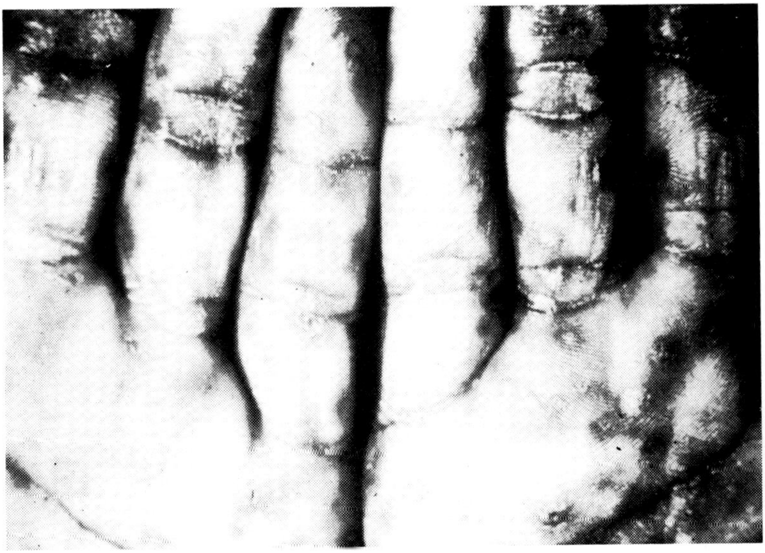

5. Secondary syphilis of the palms.

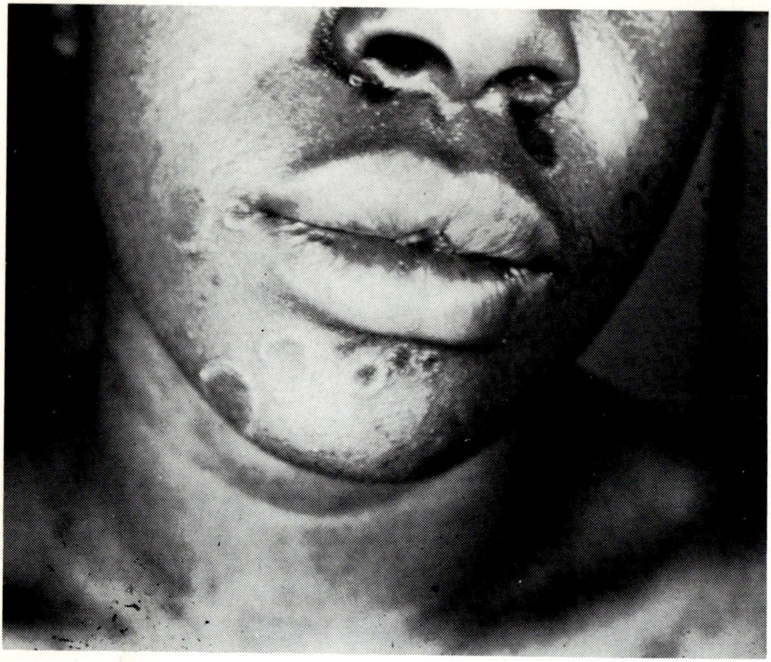

6. *Secondary syphilis. Generalized papular syphilis of the face.*

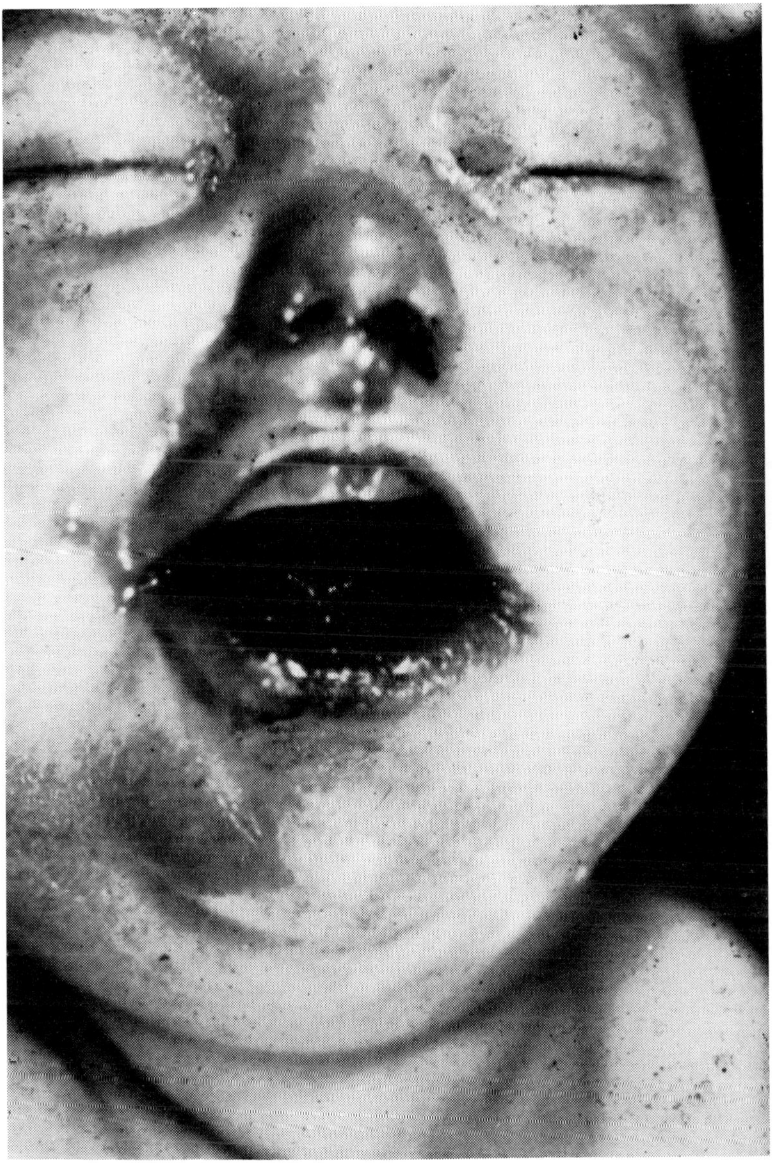

7. Congenital syphilis. Snuffles in an infant.

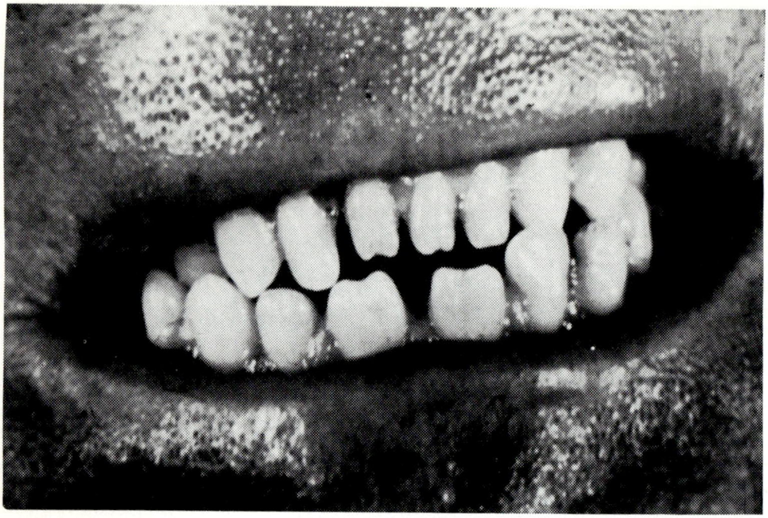

8. *Congenital syphilis. Typical Hutchinson's teeth.*

6

VENEREAL DISEASE AND VITAL STATISTICS

One of the most distracting elements involved in the writing of a medical book intended to be read primarily by other than medical personnel is the problem of *vital statistics.* To most people an aggregation of numbers is boring, and after the accumulation reaches a certain figure—usually a million—whether it be dollars or medical cases the mathematical facts lose their reality and become uninteresting to the reader. In the first place, medical statistics on dermatological and venereal cases are difficult to establish, because case histories, in the customary medical definition, are a problem to garner unless, for example, a special report or paper is being prepared. A person comes into the office with a skin ailment. Unless it needs prolonged care and attention, the number of visits to the doctor are relatively few. The case is either marked closed, or continued care persists throughout the duration of the condition (which can be lifetime), or until the patient hears of another dermatologist who has treated some other patient suffering from the same chronic skin disease and produced miraculous results. The turnover in the practice of dermatology is possibly the highest in all fields of medicine. I am also convinced that part of the difficulty in obtaining statistical facts regarding venereal disease is primarily due to the nature of the disease and the propensity to induce and perpetuate secrecy between patient and doctor.

The increase in the incidence of VD is, of course, the primary reason for writing this book. The gonorrhea increase has been going on long enough to be far beyond any chance of error or the possibility of excuse and, today, the same thing is happening with syphilis. To make this point emphatic I would like to give the reader some astounding figures to study, with their interpretation to be tempered by a degree of skepticism attendant on the scientific and statistical evaluation of the nature of the beast of VD.

The figures do lie—even as bad as they are, they are not and could not possibly be the truth and the whole truth! Under the present method of reporting cases of venereal disease, we are thwarted before we begin. My stand on the matter is not taken as a doctor practicing in Los Angeles County, where a high percentage of venereal disease is recorded—high enough to be declared of epidemic proportions—but, rather, it is taken from the world point of view, as observed through the World Health Organization, a clearing house for all countries affiliated with the organization. The problem is basically that all available statistics are based on cases reported through local public health authorities, whether it be in Copenhagen or in Los Angeles. In truth, however, the number of reported cases bears little resemblance to the actual number of cases.

All reported disease statistics are subject to error, but VD statistics suffer more than others. Perhaps doctors and patients alike are guilty of playing ostrich, but there are many other logical routes of confusion: Many people with reportable diseases do not always reach a clinic or a doctor, or may go undiagnosed or misdiagnosed. There is both underreporting—cases missed—and overreporting—cases of mistaken diagnosis. As venereal disease becomes more prevalent, the statistics tend to level off for obvious reasons, i.e., the doctor is obliged to report the scientifically confirmed cases which might have been missed in the first instance and wrongly reported in the case of the mistaken diagnosis. The occurrence of many diseases—such as the bubonic plague—have, through the centuries, been hidden by the authorities, because the knowledge was "bad for business." Cholera outbreaks have recently been concealed in areas where the big business of tourism might be affected. Yet we do know that infectious diseases, when properly reported to health authorities and properly placed under care, can be controlled. Perhaps no better example of this exists than in the case of polio. The admission of epidemics in isolated locales helped to create a public demand for the discovery of a vaccine. When Dr. Jonas Salk discovered a vaccine which was accepted, the public responded and the vaccination of masses of people—children and adults alike—practically made polio a disappearing disease. Today, even a suggestion of a mild outbreak receives immediate attention as to quarantine, vaccination, and medical care.

Why doesn't this attitude exist in VD?

The crux of the matter is the stigma that still clings to VD, somewhat similar to the stigma attached to leprosy for many centuries. We must face up to the fact of VD and accept it on a purely medical plane, rather than on a moral or social one.

In the case of gonorrhea, our vital statistics are misleading because of the lack of a simple diagnostic test by which to identify the infection—especially among women and homosexual victims. We presume that a certain amount of gonorrhea exists among women prostitutes and women prisoners, yet the statistical evidence is not superficially seen, and not until the disease is well established do we have any proof of our speculations. In addition, there are many cases of gonorrhea that are treated perfunctorily and go unreported. In order the better to understand the ratio of statistics in regard to VD, let us take the case of "X," traveling across the country on business. He is alone and feels the need for sexual companionship. He goes to a bar, has a few drinks, and makes a contact. Within a week, he develops symptoms of gonorrhea. He is, in the meanwhile, many cities and many miles away from his source of contact. In fact, he is not even certain of the name of the woman who was the source of his infection. And even if he were, what good would it do—a thousand miles apart? He takes his dosage of penicillin and hopes for the best. Meanwhile, in that week's interim, how many people did he infect and how many will he inform? The chances are great that he infected others and remote that he informed anyone.

On the other hand, if "X" contracts syphilis and does not have the good fortune to have a chancre appear within three weeks but only consults a doctor when he gets the secondary manifestations (even then there is some doubt until his tests prove to be positive), he might have been traveling about the countryside indulging in his sexual needs and transmitting the disease which, in turn, is also being transmitted arithmetically.

What is the solution? The use of the condom in the male? I doubt if this would receive enthusiastic support today, either by male or female. Abstinence? This, too, is an unrealistic approach. What, then, is the answer?

The sad truth is that we do not have a positive answer to the problem of the Venus dilemma.

Certainly if, in order to obtain the actual vital information necessary for control of an infectious disease we were to be turned into a police state, where the sanctuary of the most private emotions is invaded, we would be in a bad way both as individuals and as a conglomerate society.

In our statistical data, locally and around the world, syphilis and gonorrhea are outranked in incidence as infectious diseases only by the common cold. However, while venereal disease is not No. 1 among the so-called reportable communicable diseases, the number of new cases exceeds that of strep throat, scarlet fever, measles, mumps, hepatitis, and tuberculosis combined. Nineteen seventy-two saw 624,000 new cases of gonorrhea in the United States and, considering that for every case reported four remained unreported, the real figure is nearer two million. For syphilis, which, when untreated, may lead to insanity and death, the figures are even more disturbing. Today, there are at least one-half million Americans with untreated syphilis, and the projected year's increase will include 85,000 new cases. The number of new syphilis cases currently reported for 1972 represents an increase of 16 percent over last year, and the biggest increase in two decades.

VD seems to strike hardest in the cities, where there are at least twelve cases of syphilis for every 100,000 persons. Nationwide, Newark, New Jersey, ranks first among the cities, with 124 syphilitics per 100,000 persons, followed by Atlanta, Georgia, and San Francisco, California. For gonorrhea, the case rate nationally is 308 per 100,000 of the population. In the Atlanta area, the incidence of gonorrhea is an astronomical 2,510 per 100,000; in San Francisco 2,067. And in Los Angeles in the year 1972, 6 percent of the women having babies at a major city hospital were infected with gonorrhea.

VD is particularly rampant among young Americans. At least one in 5 persons with gonorrhea is under 20 years of age. Last year, more than 5,000 cases were found among youngsters between 10 and 14, and 2,000 cases among children under 9 years of age. "The probability that a person will acquire VD by the time he's about 25 is about 50 percent," says a former chief of the Los Angeles County Venereal Disease Control Division.

Of course a major problem in the treatment of gonorrhea is that the gonococci—like the staphylococci that plague U.S. hospitals—have become increasingly resistant to penicillin. The standard amount needed to effect a cure has increased during the last 25 years from 150,000 units to 2.4 million units or more per person. Even after massive doses, many cases remain uncured, and the possibility of dangerous allergic drug reaction is ever present.

In the world picture, the story of VD parallels that of the facts in the United States, although the United States leads many countries in statistical incidence. This may be due to the fact that, despite our shortcomings, we seem to have a better grasp on our control program than other countries, but the percentages are very close. At any rate, none of the statistics available would give pause for complacency.

There are certain facts of interest, however, in statistics procured from the World Health Organization which indicate that, in areas from which yaws and bejel have been cleared, such as Yugoslavia and parts of Africa, syphilis is now appearing and on the increase.

In the Soviet Union and in China, which represent something like one-quarter of the population of the earth, the statistics that have been procured are confusing. In Russia, the figures under the czars were much lower than those following the revolution, due, no doubt, to the number of unregistered VD patients treated in private practice and to the number untreated and undiagnosed; in the figures available on gonorrhea, the overall ratio of males to females would suggest that much of the existing gonorrhea in Russian women has gone undiagnosed. Reports on the clinical aspects of both syphilis and gonorrhea appear in Soviet technical literature. The general impression obtained from reading this literature would indicate that the USSR may be somewhat, if not considerably, ahead in VD control, but in spite of its authoritarian medical care, it has come nowhere near reaching a point of abolishing VD. The plea relative to gonorrhea is that "new techniques (for example, immunization, if that can be achieved) are required."

In China, to date, we have no World Health Organization statistics at all. However, we have some available literature from two not unbiased Western observers, Edgar Snow and

Felix Greene. Earlier in the history of VD, it appears that all the commoner forms existed in China from very ancient times. We have every reason to believe that syphilis and gonorrhea both flourished there before the revolution, especially in the coastal cities where prostitution was rife. By 1960, according to Snow and Greene, VD had been virtually conquered in China. George Hatem, M.D., an American-born (Buffalo, N.Y.) doctor of Syrian ancestry who traveled to China in 1930, settled there permanently, and is known throughout China by his Chinese name, Ma Hai-Teh. He was chief of the Institute of Venereology and Skin Diseases in Peking and occupied this post during a successful national war against syphilis and gonorrhea. When this campaign was presumably completed, he became a deputy director concentrating on malaria and skin diseases. How did Dr. Ma accomplish this miracle? According to an English surgeon, Dr. Joshua S. Horn, who has written of his fifteen years' experience as a doctor in China and tells of the "conquest of syphilis," "active venereal disease has been completely eradicated from most areas and completely controlled throughout China."

> The criteria for community cure were strict. They included the finding and treatment of all existing cases, a total absence of new cases appearing in the community, disappearance of congenital syphilis in new-born babies, and normal pregnancies and pregnancy outcomes in previously treated mothers. When these criteria had been fulfilled and maintained for five years, the community was considered to be cured.

In addition, Dr. Horn supplies us with the following statistical information.

> In Peking it is impossible to find active syphilitic lesions to demonstrate to medical students. A gen-

> eration of doctors is growing up in China with no direct experience of syphilis, but this is of little consequence because the disease will never return.
>
> At a conference held in the Research Institute of Dermatology and Venereal Disease in the Chinese Academy of Medical Sciences in January 1956, specialists from eight major cities reported that a total of only 28 cases of infectious syphilis had been discovered in the four years 1952-1955. An investigation of infectious syphilis in seven major cities between 1960 and 1964 showed that by the end of this period, the rate of early syphilis was less than twenty cases per hundred million of population per year . . . that is, it had very nearly reached the point of extinction.

This report, whether prejudiced or not, does give some indication that perhaps we have more to learn medically from the Chinese than the present vogue of *acupuncture.* Obviously, the technique employed is that of a medical blitz. Would it be possible or practical to carry out such a program in the United States?

Yes, if we gave every case of infectious VD that came to notice the full epidemiological shock treatment, and made the case noninfectious, we could possibly get some strong foothold in the control of VD. Our problem is of controlling VD in a free population as we discovered when Prohibition created more problems than it solved.

Despite the discouraging statistical data on VD, there is some satisfaction in the figures available on the minor venereal diseases. Most of these have declined sharply in the United States in the past decade. Granuloma inguinale (or granuloma venereum) is caused by a bacterium that produces little bumps that turn into raw, oozing masses of tissue spreading from the groin over the genitals and buttocks. Likewise, lymphogranuloma venereum, which is the only venereal disease caused by a virus, is recognized by a lump, or bubo, the size of an egg which appears in the groin some three weeks following exposure. Both are rarely seen outside the black population of the southeastern states. Contrary to most popular belief, these diseases can be treated with sulfa drugs or antibiotics. Including the chancroid, the third minor venereal disease, the cases of these instances of VD continue to be on the decline.

All our statistics thus far compiled merely show numbers, not people with emotions who are involved in the diseases. We look at the statistics and ask: "Who gets VD?"

The young. The middle-aged. Even the very old. (In France a recent case of syphilis newly contracted was reported on a ninety-one-year-old man.) Streetwalkers. (Call girls are less prone to get involved with disease because they represent a higher economic and educational level and, since sex is their occupation, they usually are rather well informed on the subject.) Homosexuals. Heterosexuals. People on drugs. People who are ignorant and do not bother to become informed. The lazy. The careless. And above all, people who don't care, either about themselves or about anyone else. This group constitutes the great majority of statistical numbers turned into human beings with whom we have to deal. It is not an easy task.

7

THE COMPANY YOU KEEP

The arch-villains of our book on VD are obviously the spirochete of syphilis and the gonococcus of gonorrhea.

Thanks to the great microbiologists of years past, there finally emerged a realization that many diseases were caused by minute organisms, invisible to the human eye but visible under the microscope. These could be isolated, and men of science could obtain some crude knowledge of their physical identity. The hysteria which followed the discovery of the germ theory almost blanketed the theory of God's revenge upon man for his earthly sexual misdeeds. Despite writings on the bacillus of syphilis, it was not until almost at the end of the nineteenth century that the works of Fritz Schaudinn and Erich Hoffman announced the discovery of the *Trepo nema pallidum,* a spirillum, and science admitted that the cause of syphilis was known, fingered, and isolated.

As we have seen, the cornering of *T. pallidum* led to many attempts to apprehend it, until the discovery of penicillin, when the world sat back with ease in the knowledge that the villain was now incarcerated with proper diagnosis and treatment. But syphilis was not to be that easily eliminated as one of the frightening specters of mankind. The very specific for the disease became the undercover agent that postponed the important diagnosis until too late, and the specific often masked the affliction because of the common and routine use of antibiotics. Obviously until some further discovery of a preventative vaccine such as is administered in smallpox, the *Treponema pallidum* will continue to rear its ugly head.

In the case of gonorrhea, we are aware that the disease is now out of control and, in some areas pandemic, according to Dr. K. Kiraly, chief of communicable diseases of the World Health Organization. One of the chief causes of the uncontrolled worldwide rise in venereal diseases is population movement. More than 6 million European workers have emigrated from their homes and more than 125 million tourists visit Europe yearly to spread the epidemic. Obviously international surveillance of venereal diseases needs strengthening.

It is not with a casual eye that we note the epidemic course of VD and the periods in history in which these scourges have occurred. The route of epidemic travel of VD has followed on the heels of warfare, the uprooting and mixing of strange people in strange lands. Man, lost without the anchor and support of the place of his roots, in many instances seeks out numerous sexual contacts, contacts made easy by a prevailing attitude of sexual freedom and permissiveness. Spurred by fear and a lack of inner security, he is driven into periods of deep depression. In this period of neglect and despair, he seeks out and beyond himself, and in his carelessness, he brings upon himself the disease that appears to the unscientific mind to be the punishment of an angry God. It is in these times of population mobility coupled with stress and man's loss of identity that we find such epidemics of VD as we are experiencing today. The irony lies in the fact that the very science that brought us electronics and to the truth about the origin of VD also brought new horrifying methods of warfare and perpetuated the Venus dilemma. Numerologists, astrologers, palmists and a variety of Eastern sects have sprung up to fill the gap of uncertainties. It is little wonder that man has again turned to the faith-healers who, with added glamour and TV coverage, have resorted to the old evangelistic hawking, "The wages of sin is death!" If science could not control syphilis which we were certain it had conquered, what hope is there for the cure of cancer, heart ailments, muscular dystrophy and other dread diseases? Despite our scientific progress we appear to be behind the eight-ball. The physician is too often bypassed in the do-it-yourself school of action where one soon learns that a little learning is a dangerous thing.

That VD is contagious is one factor with which we have to contend in our efforts at control, but the method of its transference—through the sexual organs—is a second and more difficult factor. This factor is loaded with emotion, both in origin and development, and eventually in treatment and control. In and out of our culture we can trace the story of VD in all forms of human expression—writing, painting, sculpting. As man has traveled and evolved, so has the story of VD. The disease is of man and with man and is part and parcel of his sexual dilemma.

The impact of VD upon mankind is reflected in many of the writings which have helped create the history of man including the Bible. In Genesis 12:17, "And the Lord plagued Pharoah and his house with a great plague because of Sarah, Abraham's wife"; in Genesis 20:17-18, "So Abraham prayed unto God: and God healed Abimelech and his wife and maidservants; and they bare children. For the Lord had fast closed up all the wombs of the house of Abimelech, because of Sarah, Abraham's wife."

In the section describing sterility in Abimelech's house, we recognize the presence of VD. Bertrand Russell, one of the great modern philosophers, wrote a letter to Colette, the famous French novelist, in which appeared the following caustic comment on the lines quoted from Genesis.

> What a queer work the Bible is! Abraham who is the pattern of all virtues twice over, when he is going abroad says to his wife: "Sarah, my dear, you are a very good-looking person and the King is very likely to fall in love with you. If he thinks I am your husband, he will put me to death, so as to be able to marry you; so you should travel as my sister—which you are, by the way." On each occasion, the King does fall in love with her, takes her into his harem, and gets diseased in consequence so he returns her to Abraham. Meanwhile Abraham has a child by the maidservant whom Sarah dismisses into the wilderness with the newborn infant without Abraham objecting. Rum tale!

The Book of Leviticus is full of diseases that can be identified as VD. There is much detail as to sanitation and cleanliness, and the clear allusion to the connection between VD and copulation. One wit has traced the belief that VD could be contracted from toilet seats to Leviticus: 15:4 ". . . everything, whereon he sitteth, shall be unclean."

Biblical plagues of syphilis have been construed from the plagues of Egypt and Moab. In Deuteronomy, the words of Moses announce the rewards of disobedience to the laws of sexual sanitation.

> The Lord will smite thee with the botch of Egypt, and with the emerods, and with the scab, and with the itch whereof thou canst be healed. . . . And, the Lord shall smite thee with madness, and blindness, and astonishment of heart. . . . The Lord shall smite thee in the knees,

> and in the legs, with a sore botch that cannot be healed, from the sole of thy feet to the top of thy head. . . . Then the Lord will make thy plagues wonderful, and the plagues of thy seed, even great plagues, and of long continuance, and sore sickness. . . .

How are these plagues of early epidemics explained? When the children of Israel departed from their God Jehovah, and began to worship Baal instead. Accordingly, "The people began to commit whoredom with the daughters of Moab." Baal-worship also included fertility rites to which we have already referred.

So constant are the epidemics of recognizable venereal disease throughout early biblical history that the French syphilologist, Buret, wittily, suggested a rewrite of the first sentence of the Bible to read: "In the beginning God created the heaven, the earth, man, and VD."

In the works of the Roman historians we find repeated references to VD, often associated with homosexuality which was rampant at the zenith of Roman culture. VD in the male is often located in the anus as the result of pederasty. We are told by Catullus of Julius Caesar and his pederast, Mamurii, both of whom contracted a disease whose masked spots left stains upon their bodies that would not disappear, both being infected together in the same bed. Throughout Roman literature there are many references to physical impairments that must have been the "shining pustules" of syphilis, the "malignant ulcer" that comes from kissing, the "mournful diseases of the chin" (mentraga).

Surely the "morbus indecens" is syphilis for the Romans and, in the ruins of Pompeii which was destroyed by Vesuvius in 79 AD and rediscovered in 1775, there are innumerable inscriptions alluding to VD, one written in a brothel stating, "The most beautiful women of that establishment had the disease capable of producing ulcers."

As the disease spread throughout Europe we find the vagabond poet, Francois Villon, writing his ballads and singing of the curse of VD.

In sublimate whereof men stand in dread;
In sweat from navels of the live adders—whew!
In blood, in basins drying and all dead
For leeches use beneath the full moon—phew!
Some being black, some green in chives; in spew
Of chancre sores and those filthy crocks
Where nurses wash the blood from invalid's smocks;
In little baths the love girls lie beside
(Who knows them not, knows naught of stews, by cocks!)
Let envious tongues be fricasseed and fried.

In *Gargantua,* Rabelais, who wrote during the great epidemic of the fifteenth century, included this in the introduction: "Most illustrious drinkers, and you, most precious Syphilitics." And the demise of Gargantua is recorded thus:

And he died in the year fourteen-twenty,
Of the syphilis, which he had a-plenty.

By the time William Shakespeare appeared on the scene, VD was commonplace and he used it to his advantage as a dramatic theme as many modern playwrights have used alcoholism. Shakespeare left us marvelous and wonderful descriptions of skin diseases. For example, in *Much Ado About Nothing,* Act 3, Scene 3, Borachio and Conrade: "Here, man I am at thy elbow." Borachio: "Mass, and my elbow itched; as if there would be a scab follow." Thus, in a few words Shakespeare reveals not only the contagious nature of scabies, but its typical location as well.

Shakespeare alludes to VD almost exclusively as syphilis. So many facts and facets of the disease have been investigated in his plays, that some students have reckoned that the poet himself was afflicted with the disease. As we know, Shakespeare was a genius who acquainted himself with everything surrounding him and the life he wrote about—the intimate journals of the historical lives of kings and queens acting out their destinies in the company of soldiers, sailors, serving people, adventurers and even the inhabitants of the new world of Columbus's discovery (Caliban, of *The Tempest*). Since he wrote prolifically on all the subjects he observed, it is not strange that he should write of syphilis which was all around him.

Modern authors could do well to read the master properly and learn there is nothing new in the sexual acts of man or woman. Shakespeare was anti-Puritan just as the age of Puritanism was descending upon England, and much of the true meaning of his words were lost until scholars penetrated and revealed their implications. Shakespeare seems to have been also well educated in the study of medicine and possibly knew as much as some of the practicing physicians of that day. Most of their knowledge was derived from the writings of Hippocrates and Galen, and the same sources were available to the bard.

Shakespeare's references to syphilis can be traced through his glancing allusions, usually veiled, which come nearest to humor. Calling it the "French Disease" which was common at that time, Shakespeare has Peter Quince in *A Midsummer Night's Dream* speak of French crowns that "have no hair at all" (referring to syphilitic baldness); in *Measure for Measure,* the comedy of sex which just brushes by tragedy, Lucio is affronted by the First Gentleman who says to him: "I had as lief be a list of an English kersey as be pil'd, as thou art pil'd, by a French velvet." Lucio responds: "I will out of thine own confession, learn to begin thy health, but whilst I live forget to drink after thee."

Bullous eruptions were a common occurrence among Shakespeare's heroes. Although he generally uses the word "blister," there are obvious different bullous conditions that must be considered. In most instances, the bullous disease is herpes simplex, as in *Romeo and Juliet* (Act 1, scene 4) "O'er ladies' lips, who straight on kisses dream, Which oft the angry Mab with blisters plagues."

On the other occasions "blisters" are used as a symptom of syphilis. During Shakespeare's time, the syphilitic infection was highly virulent, and bullous and pustular eruptions were frequently noted, as demonstrated by many contemporary documents and pictures of the epoch. Shakespeare's theater was in Winchester which, at that time, was a notorious setting for brothels, the main source of syphilitic infections. There was no doubt as to how syphilis was contracted: "Some galled goose of Winchester would hiss./ Till then I'll sweat and seek about for eases,/ And at that time bequeath you my diseases." (*Troilus and Cressida,* Act V, scene 10.)

Although there might be some confusion about what syphilis was called at that time (pox, meazel, tetter, serpigo, verole, the infinite disease, etc.) there is no doubt about the clinical manifestations and the epidemiology as described by Shakespeare. In cursing Alcibiades' girl friends, Timon, in *Timon of Athens,* gives an excellent description of the early, secondary, and late manifestations of syphilis (valid to this very day) as well as its manner of conveyance:

"This fell whore of thine/ hath in her more destruction than the sword. . . . Give them diseases leaving with thee their lust" (Act IV, scene 3). Later in the play Timon describes what happens to the lovers of Timandra: "Down with the nose–/ Down with it flat; take the bridge quite away– [obviously tertiary lues] Of him that, his particular to foresee,/ Smells from the general weal. Make curl'd-pate ruffians bald,/ And let the unscarr'd braggarts of the war/ [luetic alopecial] Derive some pain from you [the scarring lesions of tertiary syphilis] . Plague all;/ That your activity may defeat and quell/ The source of all erection."

In *Henry V* we learn something of the treatment of syphilis in Shakespeare's day when Pistol observes: "O hound of

Crete, think'st thou my spouse to get?/ No; to the 'spital go,/ And from the pow'dring tub of infamy/ Fetch forth the lazar kite of Cressid's kind,/ Doll Tearsheet, she by name, and her espouse."

'Spital is the Elizabethan name for hospital, and the "pow'dring tub" refers to the treatment with mercury by fumigation; "lazar" is somebody with a loathsome body disease. Later in the play, Pistol says: "News have I that my doll is dead i' the 'spital/ Of the malady of France."

Literary references to VD after Shakespeare became rarer in English, although some allusions can be found in the poems of John Donne, the writings of Jonathan Swift, John Milton, Robert Burns, and Lord Byron. Following the growth of puritanism, a counterthrust, in part, to the corruption of morals and politics of the times, we find VD buried in a coffin of polite but effective censorship. Again syphilis is a "dirty word," an unmentionable. VD, however, was not to be effectively silenced in the arts for too long a period, being not only a disease, but a social burden too great to be ignored. In the latter part of the nineteenth century, the Norwegian poet and playwright Henrik Ibsen (1828-1906) abandoned his medical studies and turned to writing. His plays stressed individual freedom and dealt with social and psychological themes. In the last act of *A Doll's House* (which is enjoying a stage and screen revival at the time of the writing of this book), the heroine, Nora, slams the door of her house as she leaves her husband and children; this act opened the door for the liberation of women. It was the first overt cry against Victorianism.

In 1879, Ibsen gave the world *Ghosts,* a name given by its English translator, William Archer. The play reintroduced the subject of syphilis to a startled audience, which for many years had preferred to disregard the subject and classify it as taboo. The play saw its original production in, of all places, Chicago, in 1882, when it was produced by a company of touring Danish actors in the Aurora Turner Hall. Later it was produced in London where the critics labeled it "putrid." The first audiences were as shocked by the handling of the syphilis theme as they were by the novel idea that disease and death were not the wages of sin. The leading character in the play is Osvald, the congenital syphilitic son who was infected by his father. The syphilitic father does not appear on stage, and Mrs. Alving, the mother, conforms to all the virtues of the Victorian mother. The medical information in *Ghosts* is not very authentic for our times, but the impact of a play based upon the theme of syphilis is not to be underestimated.

Twenty years later and three years before the discovery of the *Treponema pallidum,* a French play *Les Avaries,* by the journalist and dramatist Eugêne Brieux (1858-1932), (entitled *Damaged Goods* in English translations), was produced and dedicated to Alfred Fournier, after whom an institute devoted to the study of syphilis was named; a year later, Wasserman described the blood test that carries his name; and in 1910, Ehrlich reported the first authentic cure called Salvarsan, or the trial chemical number "606." The introduction reads: "I think, with you, that syphilis will become much less serious when we are able to speak openly of it without shame or fear of punishment, and when those affected by it, are aware of the suffering they may cause others, will better appreciate their duty to those others as well as to themselves."

These words written in 1907 could well be transposed to the year 1970 when syphilis again reached epidemic proportions and the public was again urged to step forth and speak openly on the subject of VD—syphilis and gonorrhea.

Damaged Goods has had an interesting literary career in the United States. It was translated by Upton Sinclair who used the material as a source of one of his books. The play opened March 14, 1913, at the Fulton Theatre in New York. It was not open to the general public, but was shown exclusively to a group called the Sociological Fund. Persons who wished to see the play bought special memberships in the fund society instead of buying tickets of admission. In spite of the restrictions placed upon it, it was a "huge success acclaimed by public, press, and pulpit as the greatest contribution ever made on the stage to the cause of humanity." It was revived in 1937 at the 48th Street Theatre in New York, and in 1941 at the Butler Davenport Theatre.

The play is medically authentic and credible up to the date of writing and in the context of current medical discoveries. The leading character is a young man who learns that he has syphilis. The doctor (who is the central character and upon whom all the medical philosophy rests) advises him not to marry, but because of commitments he has made he goes *a rebours* to the doctor's advice, marries, and produces a congenitally syphilitic child. The doctor suggests to the vengeful father-in-law that he has only escaped the boy's fate by "good luck." Once the damage has been done, the doctor recommends that the solution lies in reconciliation rather than revenge and open scandal. In the final act the doctor implies that the solution to the VD problem is abstinence, in both sexes, until marriage. This pronouncement was a call for a single standard in sexual matters, that permeated the sex etiology of the twentieth century.

Interestingly enough, as medical progress was made in the discovery of a specific cure for VD, less concern was shown in the writings of the era. One book by John Horne Burns, *The Gallery,* written in 1947, is a useful document in the literature of syphilis. One chapter "Queen Penicillin" is a gentle narrative of a reaction to being infected with syphilis by someone one deeply loves, and how it felt to be treated by an army doctor in Naples in 1944. "I don't say 'Welcome' to our hospital. You're not going to have a good time here. Our whole set-up is guaranteed to make you hate everything about us. We don't want men coming back here. See? There's no excuse for men getting VD. No excuse whatsoever. We give you treatment here, but we do it in such a way that you won't come back. . . ."

The story ends with the words of the chaplain who is afraid to shake hands with the boy. "My boy," he says, "if there were no disease in the world, there would be no decency. The fear of God! Your illness is the sign of God for God's disapproval of what you did."

It was penicillin that blacklisted VD as a subject of literary significance. VD was old hat, forgotten with Michael Arlen's *Green Hat,* atypical of the Roaring Twenties. The first contemporary playwright to invoke the ghost of VD was Tennessee Williams. In *Sweet Bird of Youth* (1959) the hero, having given his childhood sweetheart a case of gonorrhea, is thwarted in his first love affair by the girl's politician father. The boy leaves his hometown and becomes a gigolo. In the company of an aging, depraved actress, the boy returns to his hometown where he encounters his childhood sweetheart. He learns that she was forced to undergo an operation and "the knife had cut the youth out of me and left me an old, childless woman." At the end of the play, the boy pays the price of his youthful sin by being run out of town and castrated. The vengeance and wrath of a godhead descends upon the head—or more specifically the reproductive organs—of the man or woman trapped in the Venus dilemma.

Among the most vivid pieces of writing on the subject of VD handed down to us are those by Benvenuto Cellini and James Boswell. Cellini was the victim of syphilis, and Boswell of gonorrhea.

Cellini, the noted sculptor and goldsmith, whose craftsmanship has been unequaled, was also a compelling biographer of his own life and life-style. His *Autobiography* was translated into English by John Addington Symonds and is considered a literary classic. In it Cellini gives the following account of how he contracted syphilis and cared for his condition.

It is true indeed that I had got the sickness, but I believe that I caught it from that fine, young servant girl whom I was keeping when my house was robbed. The French Disease, for it remained in me dormant more than a month, before it showed itself and broke out over my whole body in one instant. It was not like what one commonly observes, but covered my flesh with certain blisters of the sizes of sex-pences, and rose-colored. The doctors would not call it the French Disease, albeit why I told them I thought it was that. I went on treating myself by their methods, but derived no benefit. At last, then, I resolved on taking the wood [guaiac] against the advice of the first physician in Rome. I took it with the most scrupulous discipline and rules of abstinence that could be thought of; and after a few days, I perceived a great amendment. The result was that at the end of fifty days I was cured and as sound as a fish in water.

But sometime later, after staying out in the marshland in winter, I fell a hundred times more ill than I had been before. I put myself once more under the doctor's orders, and attended to their directions but it grew worse. When the fever fell upon me, I resolved again on having recourse to the wood, but the doctors forbade me saying that if I took it with the fever in me, I should not have a week to live. However, I made up my mind to disobey their orders observing the same diet as I had formerly adopted, and after drinking the decoction for four days, I was wholly rid of the fever. My health improved enormously, and while I was following the cure I went on always working. . . . After fifty days my health was re-established.

> When at last, I ventured to relax my rigid diet, I found myself as wholly free from those infirmities as if I had been born again.

The first of these episodes is a good description of secondary syphilis, not remarkable for severity. The second, with clinical details lacking, might have been a recurrence, or more likely, a new infection, or even a different kind of illness; but the two periods of latency, including the one that may have followed an unnoticed chancre, support Cellini's self-diagnosis. His response to guaiac is irrelevant. In the *Autobiography,* he never mentions the disease again nor gives any symptoms which might have been late manifestations of syphilis. His indomitable will which led him to defy the diagnosis and treatment prescribed by physicians (about 1531), is indicative of his entire personality and his powerful intellect and creativity. There is also reason to believe from Cellini's accurate writing that at the time of the Great Epidemic there were relatively mild cases of syphilis as well as death-dealing cases, which is commonplace in epidemic diseases.

Details of James Boswell's gonorrhea (1740-1795) have been gleaned from his private papers which were not published until 1928. Boswell was not only the devoted biographer of Samuel Johnson whom he worshipped, even idolized; he emerges in his own memoirs as a more human and more interesting character than the enormous man whom he followed with doglike devotion. He is neither reticent nor puritanical, which is remarkable considering his Calvanistic upbringing, in discussing his own vices as well as his virtues. He records nineteen episodes of urethritis. He was first infected by a minor actress in 1760—a lass named Sally Forrest, whose fame rests, posthumously, on the fact that she was one of the first women who were listed as having passed the disease on to a man. Boswell's second encounter was with a lady named Louisa, whom Boswell sought out as a companion for a "safe winter's copulation." When Boswell discovered that he was enduring a new bout with the "clap" he upbraided poor Louisa who admitted having had the disease three years earlier, but had thought herself healthy for the last fifteen months. Silent but persistent gonorrhea in women was not suspected then. As we read the *Journals,* we see Boswell emerge as a man "trapped by forces beyond his control, his motives deeper than his insight, driven to a life of chronic anxiety, ridden by a continuing sense of guilt and need for punishment, intemperate and incontinent, impairing his manhood by courting and receiving venereal disease in expiation, and finally dying of its sequalae" (Dr. William Ober). How analagous is the story of Boswell to many victims of VD! The times and the settings have changed, but the diseases and the consequences have remained static.

Among the young geniuses who are thought to have been sacrificed on the altar of VD was the poet John Keats (1795-1821) who suffered from VD in addition to the tuberculosis from which he died. Keats, who was himself trained as a medical doctor, twice took the mercury cure for syphilis. The theory that there is a link between the raging fevers of the tubercular and the abnormal need for sexual release make Keats's case a classic. His contemporary, Franz Schubert (1795-1828), who contracted syphilis at the age of twenty-four, also received the mercury treatment and died at thirty-one from a combination of tuberculosis, syphilis, and enforced poverty. Born in the same year but surviving longer, was the German poet, Heinrich Heine, whose syphilis began at the age of twenty-four but continued with secondary and late symptoms including neurosyphilis leading to paralysis late in life. The list of authors includes such illustrious names as Charles Baudelaire, Oscar Wilde, Gustave Flaubert, Fydor Dostoevski, Alphonse Daudet, and our own Walt Whitman, whose *Leaves of Grass* immortalized the common man and exalted man's love of his fellow man. Whitman's love of his fellow man caused him to die a paralytic syphilitic. Of course, many people who are not talented and not bohemian in their outlook on life also get venereal infections, but that VD infected and affected the lives of many men of creative genius is not unusual, for the very compulsion of their talent lay in the intimacy of their emotional and sexual contacts with other human beings.

In the graphic and plastic arts, the concept of VD has been largely confined to the "fright school." It extends from the early art of pre-Columbian days to the modern use of color photography. Most scholars and students of man are acquainted with the art of Albrecht Dürer who made a well-known woodcut entitled "The Syphilitic" and wrote many letters in which he noted his dread fear of syphilis. The woodcut was used to illustrate a medical pamphlet and is not one of the gifted artist's better works. It shows the figure of a man with spots, described as ulcers but drawn as rings and shown on all parts of the body not covered by cloak, hat, and boots. The face is long and sorrowful, giving service to Fracastoro's description of the vague, characteristic melancholy of syphilis. There are spots on the extended right palm and, above the man, there is a sphere bearing the date 1484, the year of the astrological conjunction of Saturn, Jupiter, and Mars and the date of the Great Epidemic.

The work is the first among many whose subject was the dread disease. Dürer's obsession with syphilis indicated that he might have suffered from it himself. He deserted his wife after a few weeks of marriage and was known to frequent bathhouses in Strasbourg which were known to be hotbeds of infection. He did some of his finest work during the period between 1494-1503, a series entitled "Women, Death, and the Devil," of which the theme is related to syphilis. During this period he also did a famous self-portrait which tends to support the theory that the artist himself was infected. In the self-portrait, in pen and brush with white highlights, the artist depicts an abnormal left testicle which can be identified as a syphilitic fibrosis. In a later sketch, Dürer is pointing to a circled area on his abdomen. In an inscription on the drawing is written: "There on the yellow spot where my finger is pointing is where the pain is," proving that in those days patients could obtain as much medical advice from a doctor with a well-drawn sketch as by an interview with the doctor himself.

In addition to Dürer, there were other artists who painted VD in all its horror. One woodcut by Bartholomew Steber, *A Mala Franczos,* is very well known. It shows two patients, a woman sitting on a bed and a man sitting on a stool beside the bed. Both patients are marked with indistinctive spots, presumably ulcers. A doctor stands on one side seriously regarding an urn of urine and another is kneeling applying something from a jar to the patient's leg with a long spatula, indiscreetly turning the knee of the infected patient and illustrating how it was possible for a careless doctor to get the disease without sexual contact.

The other contemporary woodcut is from another book, *Tractatus de Scorra* by Grünspeck, in which an enthroned queen is shown holding a spotless baby and extending her right hand to an already crowned heir. Kneeling at her left are two supplicating women who are spotted on their exposed faces, necks, and hands. At the feet of the queen is the supine figure of a man, or possibly a corpse who is spotted with the familiar pox.

There are some seventeenth-century drawings that illustrate the treatment of syphilis and, accompanying the drawings, is the familiar lovesick song of Francois Villon: ". . . pour une joye, cent doleurs."

In the work of Hogarth, *The Harlot's Progress,* we find the great artist using words to indicate part of the subject, "Once out of the hospital our Margaret continues to ply her trade.

Do you know one of these creatures who has not had the clap? Our Margaret had it. Elixirs, pills, and emetics have so exhausted her that she is tired of living and dies."

The etymology for the English word "clap" in common vernacular for gonorrhea is not definitely known, but is assumed to have descended from *clapoire,* the French for rabbit warren and house of prostitution, which, in turn, is derived from *clapier,* an Old Provençal word meaning heap of stones and rabbit warren. We see that as early as Hogarth it was in common usage.

William Blake used VD in his works of art and it is to Blake we owe the couplet:

> "Let the brothels in Paris be opened
> With many an alluring dance
> To awaken the physicians thro' the city—"
> Said the beautiful Queen of France.

Rembrandt dealt with syphilis in one of his portraits, and such renowned artists as Daumier and Cruikshank—all artists who depicted social subjects—have portrayed VD on their canvases. But the encroaching puritanism tended to push VD out of the realm of art and by the time such artists as Toulouse-Lautrec and Aubrey Beardsley, both famous for their vignettes on the ladies of the bordello, appeared public taste and social customs decreed that art about VD was uncouth. Its prevalence was well known and it slunk about the populace like a virulent ghost affecting the lives of the people amongst whom it dwelt, but there were no visible signs in the arts, mere innuendos about an evil that lurks in the lives of man. Two tragic geniuses of this period, Paul Gauguin, who fled to Tahiti and painted the beauties of the Polynesian world and brought with him the infliction of syphilis transmitting it to the native people, and Vincent Van Gogh, who frequented bordellos, contracted syphilis and was finally committed to the asylum at Arles, have left behind them magnificent works of art created in spite of the death knell of VD.

For medical purposes, the invention of the camera made photographs of lesions, chancres, and other unsightly, grisly infections available for the medical student's eye. Movies later entered the scene and many a man recalls leaving a required session on VD with a queasy stomach and a fear and distaste for sex, which fortunately did not last too long!

In briefly sketching the role VD has played in the history of man in his day-to-day living and in his works of art, we note that many are under the impression that VD is of the "common people." Actually, at one time syphilis was known as the "disease of kings," the reason being that only monarchs and men of means and leisure had time to indulge in promiscuous sexual activities. From the highest rulers it seeped to the masses where it went unattended and became the poor man's calamity. As all diseases thrive best in an atmosphere of filth and ignorance, VD is no exception and for many reasons VD often hit the poorer classes more virulently than those classes of people capable of obtaining medical help. It is interesting to observe how VD is ignored in the history books and in the private biographies of many famous people who have been afflicted. Again, because of the manner in which VD is contracted, revealing a man or woman's encounter with VD demands a deep perusal into the private life of the individual. As hero worshippers, we hate for our idols to have feet of clay, and it is with hesitation that a biographer reveals about a prominent person that he was afflicted with VD. In the tradition of VD, both the Colonel's lady and Judy O'Grady have the same proclivity if exposed. The impact of VD is serious regardless of the status of the victim, but the dramatic consequences resulting from a blocked urethra in gonorrhea or syphilitic insanity in an absolute monarch or a creative genius like Nietzche, whose thought influenced the makers of history, cannot be underestimated.

There is no doubt that the spirochete and the gonococcus have inflicted untold suffering during the centuries upon millions of people.

Most of the names of famous victims of VD are taken from post-mortem diagnoses, so well concealed were the facts at the time the person was alive. In actuality, it would appear that Christopher Columbus himself was a victim of the disease he is credited with bringing to Europe. Thomas Parran, M.D., the American authority on syphilis, says that Columbus undoubtedly died from syphilis. "He began to hear voices and regard himself as an Ambassador of God." Perhaps it was for this reason that he was bound in chains and sent back to Spain by Bobadilla, the newly appointed governor of the islands.

Despite his illness, Columbus made the last voyage and returned in 1504 so ill that he had to be carried ashore. With his entire body dropsical, from the chest downwards, as if there were an injury to the valves of the heart, his limbs paralyzed, and his brain affected—all symptoms of late, fatal syphilis—he died on May 20, 1508.

Dr. Parran tells us that Charles VIII of France, the besieger of Naples, probably also had syphilis. His condition is suggested by the death of his four children in infancy, the last of the direct Valois dynasty. That Francis I was a syphilitic is recorded by Rabelais.

> In the year fifteen forty-seven
> Francis died at Rambouillet
> Of the pox he had.

The fate of France is illustrated by Dr. Parran as an example of what happens to a nation when its absolute ruler is governed by the impulses of irritable inconsistency and the delusions of grandeur which accompany one type of late syphilis.

Dr. Parran writes also of Henry VIII of England:

> Henry VIII of England can be cited to illustrate the effect of this disease upon the fate of a nation. Catherine of Aragon, his first wife, bore him four children, all still-born or dying immediately after birth, before the birth of her single living child, a daughter, later to reign as "Bloody Mary." Mary, herself showed many signs of the congenital infection—the face prematurely old and scarred; the thin, moth-eaten hair, the square head with the grotesquely protruding forehead, the extremely bad sight, which was probably due to interstital keratitis (scarring within the cornea of the eye). Her sudden death at the age of forty-two is supposed to have been due to a syphilitic aneurism (a "bubble" formed on the large blood vessel by the thinning of its wall).

Further evidence of Henry's syphilitic condition is his extreme cruelty in later life when he executed 3 percent of the population of London as well as most of his wives, behavior that could have been the result of paresis or syphilitic insanity.

In the letters of Frederick the Great of Prussia to Voltaire we find evidence that he was infected with gonorrhea; "I had the honor to receive, worse luck! from a certain Empress, a boiling hot piss."

Certain circumstances regarding Catherine the Great of Russia suggest that she had syphilis. Her natural son, Paul I, who succeeded her was a congenital syphilitic, having developed a saddle nose at the age of ten and being subject to fits of uncontrollable rage later. It is said that Catherine had syphilophobia and had her lovers screened through six ladies-in-waiting, "les Epreuveuses" (the testers). And it was she who founded the first VD hospital in the world in St. Petersburg.

Napoleon Bonaparte contracted gonorrhea while he was a young lieutenant in Paris and became a syphilitic during the Hundred Days following Elba.

Of the more recent monarchs, Edward VII of England (1841-1910) is known to have contracted gonorrhea and transferred it to his beautiful wife, Queen Alexandra. His nephew, Prince Alfred, died of syphilis in 1899. And the elder son of Edward VII, Albert Victor, Duke of Clarence, brother of George V, died in 1892 at the age of twenty-eight reputedly of syphilis of the brain. It is this duke who, today, is suspected of having been Jack the Ripper, the notorious London murderer. It is by the slight twist of destiny that shapes our ends that the Duke of Clarence died before he was married to his fiancée, Mary; after his death she married his brother George, who was the reigning monarch during World War I. What her fate might have been if her royal spouse had been Jack the Ripper is highly speculative.

In the same period we have the tragic story of Lord Randolph Churchill, father of Sir Winston. His children by his American wife, Jennie Jerome, were born before he was infected or during the period of latency, but the effect of the madness of his father upon the child, Winston, is now common knowledge. In this case we have an excellent example of how the disease affects the lives of all identified with the victim, whether by actually infecting them with the disease or by bestowing upon them a perpetual neurosis evidencing itself in chronic alcoholism and attendant fits of depression with an ultimate sense of futility and frustration.

American history has recently revealed that Woodrow Wilson contracted syphilis as a young man. His paralysis, which was syphilitic in origin, created a dilemma that had never before been encountered in American history and, for two years before his death, the country was ruled by Wilson's wife and his friend, Colonel House.

There is no doubt that Mussolini was a victim of both gonorrhea and syphilis. There is a record of the treatment given Il Duce in Switzerland, a treatment that was possibly effective for there were no evidences of the diseases at his death. But, the behavior pattern of delusions of grandeur and barbaric ruthlessness, although not always the results of syphilis, are characteristic of syphilitics.

Obviously the roster is mammoth. Just a glimpse is enlightening as a tract on the dilemma of VD which accompanies the sex act. Out of the suffering of the many persons who have lived nobly and given the world outbursts of genius proportionate to the magnitude of their sexual passions, there are millions more who have lived in ignomony and died unsung. Like so many victims of VD whom I have seen in my private practice, one of the effects of the diseases upon the later lives of the men and women affected is the warping of their sexual relationships. Many men become sexually impotent or resort to abnormal sexual perversions for the essential sexual release. Others become ascetic and withdraw from all sexual contacts.

The curse of ignorance has and continues to hover over VD, and the price paid by man has been more prohibitive in the restriction of talent and the destruction of genius before it is full-blown. Our only hope is to spare the creators of the future the pain that has had its source in VD by working for the eradication of venereal disease. Improving conditions that affront the dignity of man is the ultimate goal of the true humanist; and to all sufferers of VD—whether great and powerful, brilliant and bold, maniacal and ruthless, creators of art and beauty, or merely sick, anonymous slaves to disease—the continued existence of VD is a curse upon the mansions of the rich and the hovels of the poor. There is no line of demarcation in the final analysis of suffering and untimely or violently insane death.

The pervasiveness of VD and its penetration into so many areas of human life—its creative, physical, emotional, mental, and sexual aspects—has been the subject of this chapter. As an unusual sidelight, the recreational aspect is represented as well in philately: stamp collecting. It has been the custom of all nations for centuries to honor a person or recognize a particular subject by issuing a stamp. Many diseases have been singled out in this way—malaria, leprosy, smallpox, and recently, cancer. Pregnancy and maternity, whose sexual origins are undisputed, have appeared as subjects, but no group such as the World Health Organization has sponsored a stamp inspired by this most human disease of love and sex.

Not altogether neglected, however. Many names associated with VD have been honored by appearing on stamps that have become collector's items. Fracastoro, who gave syphilis its name, appears on an Italian stamp. Ambroise Paré, who first described syphilis in children and considered the proper treatment a topical administration of mercury, and who first noted the relationship between syphilis and aortic aneurysm, is engraved upon a French stamp. Jean-Alfred Fournier, who established the relationship between syphilis and tabes dorsalis and introduced bismuth in the treatment of syphilis, was honored on a French stamp—the sale of which was used to raise funds to fight venereal disease! Hideyo Noguchi who proved that *Treponema pallidum* was the cause of syphilis is on a stamp issued by Japan. (However the discoverers of *Treponema pallidum,* Fritz Schaudinn and Erich Hoffman, have not yet been honored.) The discovery of arsephenamine of Salvarsan by Paul Erlich cause him to be immortalized upon a German stamp. Julius Wagner-Jauregg, the Austrian neurologist and psychiatrist who discovered the use of fever treatment for general paralysis in the management of syphilis of the central nervous system is envisaged on Austrian stamps as is Karl Landsteiner who introduced darkfield microscopy for the diagnosis of primary syphilis. The Belgian public-health worker, Ernest Malvolz, who contributed much to the fight against syphilis when he established the original venereal disease clinic in 1912 is the subject of a Belgian stamp.

But there still remain so many eminent names which have been neglected. Hunter, Hutchinson, Wasserman, Parran, just to mention a few. It has occurred to me in the process of writing this book, and recognizing the need for enlightenment and financial assistance in order to eradicate VD that a series of stamps might be issued—at high premium value to collectors, and with great media publicity to further the story of VD—by individual countries or by the United Nations, to alert the world of the presence of VD, and the need to conquer it—internationally. It is a thought dropped like a pebble in the ocean. Upon what shore will the cleansing wave wash up to help inaugurate a cleansing program for the eventual eradication of VD?

8
TO BE OR NOT TO BE

At this stage of the game, the number-one question in regard to VD is that of control. How, under our political structure, is effective control possible? And how can we organize it?

First, let us study control as it is understood medically in relation to other infectious diseases. In our country, we have staged a battle against cholera, malaria, smallpox, yellow fever, typhus, polio, bubonic plague, and diphtheria—not to mention a number of "flu" epidemics. When we say "control" in regard to each of these diseases, we mean that compared with their past history as scourges, they have been effectively checked. Medically, the word control does not mean that any of these diseases can be disregarded, and that doctors across the country may fail to be alerted to any single appearance of any single one of the diseases mentioned. Control means what it suggests: that doctors be so alerted that the slightest indication of the appearance of any of these diseases that might reach epidemic proportions if unheeded, must be apprehended in the beginning. Contrary to what the lay public understands by the word control, it does not mean the elimination of the disease, although elimination is the logical ultimate goal.

The control of VD would not necessarily mean that the very last case of infection would be ferreted out and cured. It could mean a reduction to such low levels (as indicated in the Chinese report) that the proper surveillance of the few remaining patients with infectious syphilis and gonorrhea could be kept under observation until the disease was past the infectious stage. Since VD presents its greatest problem in the large cities, an outbreak could be stopped if carriers were properly checked and reported in a manner similar to that in which typhoid is controlled: When small outbreaks occur, the public health authorities are notified and are aware that the source is the drinking water or some food that has been contaminated by a carrier. An all-out alert immediately puts the situation under control and we see just how infectious diseases can be halted.

The control of infectious diseases is usually contingent upon two measures: sanitation and immunization. Sanitation was the prime agent in the control of typhus, yellow fever, typhoid, cholera, where the elimination of the carrier through means of sanitation was accomplished once science had isolated the carrier. Sanitation is the more perfect of the two measures because it eliminates the microbe before the human being is attacked. In the case of Yellow Jack, the elimination of the mosquito was the mainstay of the control.

Immunization in the form of vaccine is most dependable in viral diseases—smallpox and polio being outstanding examples—but vaccines for microbic diseases not due primarily to toxins tend to be less dependable. Venereal diseases fall into this category. So far, as we have seen, we have no vaccines against them and it is highly improbable that truly effective vaccines can be developed soon. Sanitation is not practical for control of venereal diseases because the agents of infection pass from individual to individual, and the sources of contact are usually not in the same environment for a sufficient length of time to give medical authorities any possible opportunity to confine them.

The other method of handling infectious diseases is through treatment. This is the method used with VD. Incredibly, if caught in time, both gonorrhea and syphilis are among the most easily cured of all infectious diseases. One of the most important messages of this book is that VD can be cured. That it can be constrained is also true, but that it can be cured cannot be understated. This is so of gonorrhea as well as syphilis, in spite of the resistance of gonorrhea to penicillin. The fact is that if the patient is given a dose of penicillin that doesn't work, a larger dose usually will, and if penicillin fails, there are alternative drugs. One of the most important things a patient dealing with VD must accept is that there is no limit to the amount of antibiotics the body can take. The body can and will take all the antibiotic necessary to eliminate the disease. The important factor that is overlooked is that the average patient assumes that a certain amount of penicillin will automatically cure VD. The other rules and regulations prescribed along with the antibiotic cure are usually bypassed and, as a consequence, the patient is only following the doctor's orders to a minimal degree leading to the failure of the treatment solution to VD. The infected patient simply does not follow the doctor's orders when left to exert his own free will.

If upon suspecting VD the patient would consult a doctor before there is any danger of passing the infection on to another person, the problem of VD would be cleaned up so rapidly that the mention of a "social disease" would be as dated as a bustle or a farthingale.

It was, without doubt, the discovery of penicillin and the awareness that VD could be wiped out with this drug that made the public lax, and made doctors feel that VD per se was conquered. It was the failure of the human being to assume personal responsibility for its control, immediately to seek professional help from the moment of suspected infection, and to abide by the rules prescribed by the doctor that lay the foundation for the epidemic proportions of the disease before anyone took notice.

The history of VD would seem to indicate that to have thought in terms of attempting to control it by means of treatment before the day of penicillin would have been sheer insanity. But this is not so. Endeavors were made, and the first attempt at control was naturally in the area of prostitution.

In ancient Rome, when debauchery reached an all-time high, the only concern was to "watch over the cleanliness and dress of prostitutes, and over the luxurious and comfortable fittings of the privileged houses." By the time of the Emperor Constantine in the beginning of the fourth century (306-337), harsh punitive measures to restrict prostitution were enforced, such as the confiscation of furniture, clothing, and houses, whipping and banishment. These measures, although ineffectual, were continued until the ninth century. The four centuries that followed Charlemagne were times of "great immorality." From the time of Louix IX (Saint Louis) in the thirteenth century, when it was recognized that attempts to prohibit prostitution were futile, a complete turnabout approach was made to tolerate and regulate its practice. Special neighborhoods were allotted to prostitutes. Avignon, Toulouse, and many other towns like Paris, Venice, and London had their prostitution districts, and special laws with reference to prostitutes.

When the "great pox" fell over Europe, prostitutes were the recognized carriers, and brothels the breeding houses of disease. In the fifteenth century, according to E. Lancereaux who, in 1869, published a two-volume *Treatise on Syphilis:*

> The sequestration of syphilitics was the law of that period. The rich were compelled to remain in

> their houses, the poor were driven away and threatened with death, and abandoned even by the physicians, who felt themselves unable to combat the disease. . . .

In 1496 the parliament of Paris banished all foreigners affected with "the great pox," and James IV of Scotland ruled that all syphilitics must leave Edinburgh or be branded on the cheek with the mark of the "unclean"!

In 1714, rules for sanitary regulations for a house of prostitution in Paris were firm. "The keeper of the house was required to be responsible for the sanitary condition of the women and that all, without exception, should be subjected to constant visits made by surgeons attached to the police and under the direction of a head surgeon." Even then there was a desire on the part of doctors for the establishment of public offices or special hospitals for the treatment of venereal diseases.

In 1788, an attempt was made in Denmark to provide *free* medical service for VD.

> Every person, rich or poor, suffering from a venereal disease should receive free medical advice, free medicine, together with free nursing when infirmaries or premises were equipped for the patient's treatment, that patients must agree to take treatment; that those who failed to do so should be punished.

The regulation failed in its purpose since the Danish government had to content itself with the voluntary submission for treatment on the part of infected persons. The result was that the government declared that, "In this way the disease will never be eradicated!"

The first dispensary for prostitutes seems to have been established in Paris in 1802. The emphasis was on women, and the punishment was severe. Each soldier with VD was required to go to the dispensary and there "Point out the woman who had infected him."

The rules and regulations for control of VD in the houses of prostitution became worldwide. In the United States, especially in the city of New Orleans which followed the Napoleonic Code, the standards of bordello rules and regulations became accepted on a national scale. The Madams moved from the renowned Storyville red-light district of the Crescent City to other American cities—St. Louis, Chicago, San Francisco—to mention only some of the larger metropolitan areas in which controlled prostitution flourished. Houses were established where the health rules of Paris, via New Orleans, prevailed.

Ironically, the woman was always the villain—or, villainess!

The interesting sidelight on the subject of VD and its involvement with the respectable members of society came in the nineteenth century, when it was commonplace for the head of the household to frequent the bed of the "tweenie" or any one of the maids who appealed to him. Very often it was the wet-nurse in attendance on his wife who had recently delivered a child—and the husband's VD, originally contracted in a bordello, was passed through menials into his own home. The idea of punishing a man who willingly transmitted syphilis or gonorrhea to a poor working woman was never considered of sufficient import to be discussed or included in any of the literature, medical or sociological, on the subject of VD control.

Control measures for infectious diseases, in general, were begun in the nineteenth century. In 1851, a First International Sanity Conference to deal primarily with cholera and plague was called in France. VD was identified with broad social issues rather than with health. Discussions of proper prophylaxis for VD took place, and a recommendation was made which constantly cropped up at the sundry international meetings occurring before World War I, when most of the nations of the world were engaged in a vast colonial expansion period: that it would be wise to distribute leaflets "which emphasized the dangers of VD to persons entering the armed forces."

The need to do something about VD became obvious during World War I, but the difficulties were almost insurmountable. Effective treatment of gonorrhea was nonexistent, and the lengthy treatment of syphilis with arsenical drugs was obviously impossible for mass use by the military. But, at least, out of this disastrous situation there followed some attempt with the League of Nations at international control by a nongovernmental group. The International Union Against the Venereal Diseases and Treponematoses (IUVDT), was created. At the time this organization was becoming concerned about drugs and treatment for merchant seamen, the United States was embarked on a political career of isolationism and was not a member of this international effort at control.

In 1932, under the auspices of the then surgeon general and the U.S. Public Health Service, a "control" group for the study of syphilis was undertaken in Tuskegee, Alabama. The study (composed of 600 men all of whom were black) was made of men who had previously contracted syphilis. The purpose of the study was to explore the long-range effects of untreated syphilis. A similar study had been conducted in Norway, and it was this project that was being used as a model. At the time of the study, penicillin had not yet been used clinically and the only treatment available was the long, taxing, dangerous and often fatal arsenical-heavy metal routine which was of doubtful efficacy, particularly for advanced syphilis. Many patients had refused it preferring to "let nature take its course." The study had to be confined to those individuals who had remained untreated. Even after penicillin was discovered to be a cure for venereal disease in 1946, the men were not offered the treatment. There is wide speculation as to how effective penicillin, administered to those suffering from syphilis in the advanced stages, might have been, but for the purpose of the "control study of the route of syphilis without medical aid," the medication was bypassed in the interests of the study.

The study was not publicized for more than two decades and, naturally, when it was revealed, there was a loud outcry about the inhumanity displayed in using uninformed humans as guinea pigs. In view of the fact that the entire group of men was black, as if no white syphilitics existed, the study was regarded as racist and the inhumanity was attributed to the white man's intrinsic lack of feeling for the black man that existed in the South.

After forty years, the project has been canceled. Free, lifetime medical care has been offered to the 114 survivors, most of whom are over seventy years of age. The results of the routine scientific study added little medical knowledge for the study of syphilis. The fact that the experiment was begun at a date when the government was making an honest attempt to study VD, a study that seemed essential because of the moralistic attitude of society toward syphilis, is one of the many unfortunate disasters that befell this attempt to control an infectious disease which is able to reach epidemic proportions in a very short time when allowed to go unchecked in a confined area.

Control studies since the discovery of penicillin have been introduced into prisons, where VD has been eradicated with the use of penicillin given to all prisoners with or without VD. In a very short time, when every new prisoner is treated for VD upon entering the prison, there is an absence of the disease. But such mass, indiscriminate treatment is not feasible on any protracted large scale or for any long period of time.

It was at this moment in the history of the control of VD that an American entered upon the scene—a physician who was as important in the study of the subject as any of other historical character. His name was Thomas J. Parran, and he was surgeon general of the U.S. Public Health Service from 1936 to 1948. It was under his guidance that the National Venereal Disease Control Act was passed on May 24, 1938.

According to Dr. Parran, there was "officially" no VD in the United States before his time. The subject was taboo in scientific societies as well as in polite society. The disease was considered an unpleasant subject and was relegated by some to the influx of immigrants from Europe bringing their filthy diseases with them, and to others as a disease that had been imported from Africa with the slaves. The general attitude of the self-identified patriot was to banish the foreigner who had brought VD to American shores. The fact that Europe had been blaming Columbus for bringing VD to the continent from his American contacts did not seem at all illogical!

Dr. Parran proposed a triple attack for the control of syphilis. These are his words:

> First, every early case must be reported, its source ascertained, and all contacts followed up to find possible infection. Second, enough money, drugs and doctors must be secured to make treatment possible for all cases; it is not in the public interest for treatment which is our most practical means of control, to be retarded or precluded by cost. Third, both public health agencies and private physicians throughout the country must be realigned to form a united front and re-educated to use scientific modern methods in their joint fight against syphilis. In addition, citizens must be informed as to the means and methods required for public protection.

For the first time, Dr. Parran introduced the important element that *early symptoms of syphilis are so subtle that, like many minor illnesses, the patient might dismiss them,* and that the *doctor, unless specifically trained to recognize the tell-tale signs, might also overlook them.* Both of these conditions were aggravated by charlatans, drug-store patent medicines, and the fact that the *early symptoms disappear without treatment.* How factual this is today!

To offset this, Dr. Parran recommended "a blood test whenever and wherever physical examinations are given."

And, it was because of Dr. Parran that blood tests before marriage became compulsory in the United States. Dr. Parran also respected the confidential rights of the patient thus doing away with one of the obstructions in the way of treatment:

> The rights of the patient are such that his name need not be reported; his initials, his date of birth, or a serial number are sufficient for purposes of record so long as he and his infected contacts continue to take treatment.

He pleaded for the rights of the patient, and pleaded that the practicing physician

> ... learn to think of syphilis scientifically as a dangerous communicable disease, which it is; rather than moralistically as a punishment for sin, which it often is not. Also we must learn that it is everyone's business. That everybody is endangered by the present status; that everybody pays for it, whether or not afflicted by the disease; that no one agency is big enough or clever enough to do everybody's job alone.

Perhaps if World War II had not intervened, syphilis might have been put under control in the United States—and this was before the days of penicillin. But World War II occurred and all controls were scattered to the winds. Then penicillin was discovered. With penicillin, surely, control could have been effected . . . and, to a degree, it was in the armed services.

What happened is the tragic story of the failure of a great drug. Labeled a miracle drug, it was used recklessly and without giving the patient any knowledge of his disease, accepting without query the miracle cure.

9

RELATED BUT NOT VENEREAL, VENEREAL BUT NOT COMMON

In my medical career, it has been my experience to spend a large part of my time in countries where diseases exist that are caused by organisms indistinguishable from the spirochete of syphilis. These diverse maladies plague many areas of the world, but for the most part, have bypassed the western urbanized communities. Because of the perpetual existence of warfare, and because our young people are constantly being moved about the face of the earth and being exposed to the strange diseases that exist in various regions, I am including these diseases in this book.

Other Treponemal Diseases

Although not venereal in origin, these diseases are caused by the Treponemas, as is syphilis, and the causative organisms are morphologically indistinguishable. They are peculiar to dark-skinned people and are usually found in tropical regions originating predominantly among children, although they are not congenital in origin. They are *yaws, pinta,* and *bejel.*

Yaws is a chronic, infectious, contagious, nonvenereal, spirochetal tropical disease caused by *Treponema pertenue.* It is characterized by an initial skin lesion, the mother yaw, mild constitutional symptoms, and later by one or more crops of multiple raspberrylike lesions of the skin.

Occasionally, later destructive lesions occur, involving the skin and the bones. Infection produces a slowly developing relative immunity. Yaws is restricted to the tropical zones where it is widespread, being especially prevalent in hot, moist, lowland countries. It is common in the West Indies, tropical America, throughout equatorial Africa, Ceylon, Malaya, Burma, Thailand, Indochina, the Philippines, Samoa, and other Pacific islands. It is also present in northern Australia, but relatively uncommon in India and in China.

For many years there has been a sharp difference of opinion as to the identity of yaws and syphilis, and the exact relationship between these two diseases is still controversial. The conservative view holds that yaws is due to an infection by a different but closely related strain of organism. It has frequently been observed that syphilis is rare or unknown among populations in which yaws is present.

There are important clinical and epidemiologic differences between the two diseases. Yaws is not a venereal disease, it is not hereditary, and is predominantly a disease of childhood. The primary lesion of yaws is almost invariably extragenital and is similar to the lesions of the secondary stage. In moist areas, however, the mother yaw may resemble a chancroid.

In colder climates yaws occur in modified forms and it does not spread when introduced into the temperate zones. The incidence is highest among native populations whose levels of personal hygiene are low, Europeans and Americans are rarely infected, and it is more common in males than in females. The spirochetes are unable to penetrate the unbroken skin and infection occurs directly through contact of cuts, abrasions, and other cutaneous lesions with an open yaw lesion on another individual or indirectly through soiling of the broken skin with contaminated material. Generally it is transmitted from person to person, although flies are regarded with suspicion, for they feed on moist lesions and could be carriers from one lesion to another. The arguments about the affinity between yaws and syphilis have endured as long and are as comprehensive as the arguments about the origin of syphilis. The history of yaws, its introduction into the slave states of the United States, and its consequent disappearance are of considerable interest both medically and sociologically, but are of no help in resolving the present status of yaws in relation to syphilis.

The prevention of yaws consists essentially in avoidance of contact with, and the adequate protection of, open infectious lesions. In areas where the disease is endemic, mass therapy constitutes an important control measure. Primary and secondary yaws respond dramatically to therapy with penicillin and arsenicals, but tertiary yaws is resistant to treatment. The criteria of the cure is the disappearance of the lesions.

Pinta is another form of treponematosis that means "painted" and refers to the characteristic change in the skin due to loss of pigment. It is also called mal del pinto, "disease of the spotted one," or carate. It was originally suspected of being of fungus origin, until the spirochete, indicating the relationship to syphilis and placing it in the type genus treponema, was isolated, first in Mexico and later in Cuba.

Pinta is the mildest of the treponematoses and is most commonly found amongst children in tropical or semitropical countries. The contact is from skin to skin in humid, tropical countries where children go naked or only partially clothed, or from mouth to skin, or mouth to finger to skin. Usually the contacts are made before the age of sexual maturity, and by puberty the disease will have become noninfectious or immunity will have developed so that sex will have nothing to do with maintaining it. Pinta is usually regarded as a rural and primitive disease and is very ancient in origin.

The symptoms of pinta are limited to the skin except for involvement of the lymph nodes. It entails no physical disability. Its main characteristic is the appearance of dry, scaly areas of skin in which there is a bluish discoloration followed by loss of pigment. These patchy, white areas are disfiguring, the more so in dark-skinned people among whom pinta is most prevalent, and its psychological consequences are most severe.

Pinta is customarily a disease of long duration. Its lesions appear in successive crops and remain infectious for many years. This continuing infectiousness depends on delayed immunity, reflecting the mildness of the entire process.

Bejel, the third of the nonvenereal treponematoses, occurs mostly among the Arabs in the deserts of Syria and Iraq. Again, there is considerable argument concerning this disease as to whether it is a form of syphilis or yaws, since it resembles the former in the frequent appearance of mucous patches and in its affinity for children.

In syphilis, yaws, pinta, bejel—the treponematoses—the etiologic agents for all the diseases are indistinguishable from one another. The occurrence of the initial lesion varies. The susceptibility of man to the treponematoses is universal. The transmission is customarily person to person, but only in the case of syphilis is the disease venereal in origin. The distribution of syphilis is worldwide; yaws and bejel are endemic, rural, focal, but widespread in tropical areas, in primitive settings; pinta is endemic, rural, focal, in underdeveloped areas, tropical America.

Venereal, But Not Common

In our study of VD, we must glance at the diseases that are considered venereal but are not regarded in the same category as the arch-villains syphilis and gonorrhea. It is nevertheless quite true that such diseases, when contracted, can be just as frightening to the individual as either of the two major diseases. Since syphilis is the most important cause of infectious genital ulcers, *all ulcerated lesions of the genitalia should be considered syphilitic in origin until proven otherwise by repeated darkfield examinations and serologic tests for syphilis.* When syphilis is excluded, accurate diagnosis and appropriate treatment for these diseases can be pursued.

Chancroid, or soft chancre, is characterized by lesions that begin as small blisters or pustules, and rupture leaving well-circumscribed, painful, soft ulcers. The base of the ulcer is often covered by a dirty, grayish film. The lesions are usually multiple, and they vary in size from small ulcers to large gangrenous craters. The sores of chancroid are accompanied by swollen lymph glands in the groin, usually on one side. Smears of the excretion taken from the undermined edges of the ulcers will show short, Gram-negative bacilli which often appear in small clusters like "schools of fish." Unfortunately, similar patterns may be seen in other bacterially infected ulcers. Once diagnosed, chancroid responds to treatment with sulfa drugs or antibiotics.

Granuloma inguinale usually presents itself as raised, beefy red granulation tissue. The lesions are usually quite clean in appearance, unless secondary bacterial infection is present which produces in addition a sour and oddly pungent odor. Pseudobuboes may be present. These consist of subcutaneous swellings rather than actual enlargement of the lymph nodes. Granuloma inguinale is often present around the anus. Antibiotics are the drug of choice. The incidence in the United States reports an 8 to 1 ratio of cases in blacks to whites.

Lymphogranuloma venereum (LGV) usually presents to the physician an enlargement and/or suppuration of the regional lymph nodes called buboes. Because of these lesions, the condition is often erroneously referred to as "blue balls." The disease is due to the LGV agent, a large virus, and is more common in tropical and subtropical climates. A primary lesion in the genitals does not occur except rarely, and is asymptomatic and quite transient. The subsequent inguinal lymphadenopathy is usually an elongated mass with the long axis parallel to and on either side of the fold of the groin creating a characteristic sign. Areas of fluctuation can often be palpated. These should be aspirated with an 18-gauge needle to prevent spontaneous drainage and the formation of a draining fistula. The diagnosis can only be confirmed by special tests. LGV usually responds well to treatment with tetracycline or sulfa drugs. Bedrest and aspiration may speed recovery. Rectal stricture is very common in females because of the involvement of the perirectal lymph glands.

Common, But Not Necessarily Venereal

Herpes virus. As venereal diseases go, genital herpes virus infection is strictly minor league. To most people the herpes virus infection is a common cold sore, usually appearing on the lip, but today genital herpes virus infection trails gonorrhea as the second most commonplace venereal disease. Usually the patient comes to the doctor because he believes the blister to be either syphilis or gonorrhea. Besides causing pain, secondary infection, and temporary disability, HSV-2 infection has an epidemiology pattern similar (in women) to cervical cancer. Unfortunately, there is often no clinical evidence that the sexual partner is carrying the virus. At the University of Florida College of Medicine, a study was recently made of 263 men from a wide range of social and economic groups. Thirty-nine, none of whom had a history of active genital herpes, were found to carry the virus in their genitourinary tract.

Until recently, there was no really effective treatment for herpes virus infections but there now exist several promising techniques. Painting the herpes simplex sores with various dyes and then exposing them to fluorescent tubes or even incandescent lights cut the healing time by 50 percent. And the application of ordinary ether or chloroform will clear up herpes sores in as little as two days, apparently by altering the virus so as to make it more vulnerable to the body's natural defenses. The new antiviral drug, isoprinosine, has also been used effectively. Isoprinosine, which is yet to be approved for use in this country, is administered orally and seems to bolster the body's immune response to the virus. It has stopped progression of the disease and initiated healing within forty-eight hours. So far, however, there has been no oral drug discovered which will prevent herpes infection, although a vaccine developed against herpesvirus 1 is gaining wide respectability.

Two types of herpes simplex generally attack different and sharply defined areas of the body. Doctors believe that nearly everybody carries the herpesvirus somewhere in the body, probably in the nerve tissue. In most people the virus remains docile or dormant. But sometimes it becomes active, usually during a cold or a fever, after a sunburn or other exposure, or as a result of nervous tension. The result is usually cold sores or fever blisters, unpleasant but rarely harmful eruptions that often recur in the same place, on the lips or the nose or chin.

The variant virus, herpes simplex type 11, usually attacks below the waist. It causes tender clusters or blisters or sores on the thighs, buttocks, and genitals. Unlike the herpesvirus 1 which strikes indiscriminately, type 11 appears to exercise moral judgment, tending to afflict the sexually promiscuous. It is prevalent among teenagers, young adults, and prostitutes, male and female, but it is rare in children and celibate women.

At the moment of this writing, Dr. Albert Sabin has announced his theory of a link between the herpes simplex virus and the virus causing cancer of the lip, the cervix, and those mucous areas where herpes abounds. In addition, as in the case of gonorrhea, it has been discovered that mothers with genital herpes can pass the virus off to their offspring who may develop skin lesions and internal infections. Again, the virus may be responsible for more serious illnesses in the carriers themselves, since the type 11 virus particles have been found to transform normal animal cells into cancerous ones in test tubes. Genetic substances of herpes virus have been isolated from the cells of women with cervical cancer, and in a test group of 900 women at Emory University known to have had genital herpes (comparing them with 600 women who have not had the infection) it was shown that evidence of cervical cancer was eight times higher in the first group than in the second.

But regardless of the grim spectacle of the correlation of the simple cold sore to cancer, the victim of herpes simplex can suffer pain and embarrassment which, for untreated sores, can last interminably.

Nongonococcal urethritis. This is not a specific disease. It may be traced to any one of a number of causative organisms; frequently it is impossible to determine its true etiology. As gonorrhea is commonly known as the "clap," nongonococcal urethritis is usually recognized by the lay person as the "gleet." Smears show pus and epithelial cells, but no organisms can be determined on culture.

Sexual intercourse is probably the principal mode of transmission. Excessive sexual activity and heavy drinking are believed to be precipitating factors.

Discomfort and pain in the urethra, glans, testicles, perineum, and inguinal regions are common complaints. The burning sensation in urinating associated with gonorrhea is seldom found, but pruritus is a common complaint in addition to initiating urination.

Treatment consists of antibiotic therapy, but for resistant cases a complete urologic evaluation is advised.

While bacillus Calmette-Guerin vaccination remains one of the most hopeful experimental approaches to cancer, BCG injections are also gaining attention as a treatment for recurrent genital herpes. It is conceivable that this form of immuno-therapy may have a definite place in the treatment of resistant cases.

Venereal warts. The course of the infection of warts is erratic; it may persist as a single lesion or satellite lesions may develop by autoinoculation. Venereal warts or "moist" warts are so named because they are found in the anogenital region and may simulate syphilitic condylomas. They become exuberant and may coalesce to form sizable plaques. Scattered warts may be seen in the vagina or rectum, and may serve to "seed" the skin around the orifice. None of the presently available methods of treatment is entirely satisfactory. Although warts can be removed by a variety of methods, the virus often remains and the warts recur. When performed by a doctor, freezing with liquid nitrogen may produce satisfactory results. Surgical excision is sometimes resorted to leaving painful scars. Podophyllin benzoin tincture applied at weekly intervals is effective in a reasonable percentage of anogenital warts, but occasional hypersensitivity is encountered. The origin is viral and commonplace and highly contagious.

Scabies is a transmissable parasitic skin infection, characterized by superficial burrows, intense pruritus and secondary inflammatory changes. Scabies is caused by the itch mite seldom seen in good hygienic environments. However, during war and dislocation, it may come to epidemic proportions. The impregnated female mite burrows into the stratum corneum and deposits her eggs along the tunnel. The larvae hatch within a few days and tend to congregate around hair follicles. Scabies is transmitted readily, often through an entire family, by intimate contact with an infected individual, and it may spread by venereal contact.

Itching always occurs, and is most intense, at night. The inflammatory lesions occur on the hands, the genitals of men, about the nipples of the breasts of women, the elbows, along the belt line, and on the lower buttocks. The face is not involved, and the characteristic initial lesion is the burrow—appearing as a fine, wavy, dark line varying in length from a few millimeters to a centimeter, with a minute papule at its open end. A positive diagnosis may be made by removing the parasite from a burrow with a needle. When the disease has persisted for several weeks, secondary lesions (scratch dermatitis, eczema, or superimposed bacterial infection) can confuse the diagnosis. Standard treatment includes a prolonged hot bath with particular attention to vigorous cleansing of the areas of predilection. Application of 25 percent benzyl benzoate emulsion or other parasiticide to the *entire* wetskin surface with a second application the following morning. Further applications should be avoided for they may result in an irritant contact dermatitis. Laundering of underclothing plus dry cleaning of outer garments is mandatory. If scratch or contact dermatitis occurs, calamine lotion is effective. Psychoneurotic patients may develop a persistent parasitophobia after scabies. Patients showing such tendencies should not be informed of the diagnosis, or should be reassured of the effectiveness of the cure.

As Alice discovered wandering through Wonderland, one of the most difficult things in communication was a single word with two or more meanings. The use of the word venereal in relation to diseases other than syphilis or gonorrhea is such a word. Although the reason might be clear and logical to the doctor, to the patient the word, *venereal,* is fraught with fear, embarrassment, and even shame, because the diseases involved in the genital regions are associated with sex and frequently the disastrous sequalae of syphilis or gonorrhea. Syphilis has been designated as the "great imitator" because it can mimic so many diseases. It would be impossible to tabulate in this book a list of such diseases or to discuss in detail their differential diagnosis. However, a constant awareness of syphilis on the part of the physician is of the greatest value in coming to an accurate diagnosis of the disease. It is in this sphere that the syphilologist should be consulted. While syphilis may imitate the disease, fine details of the morphologic changes in the skin make clinical recognition possible and, in many instances, paramount. These diseases I have termed the "gay deceivers." For the most part they occur in the anogenital region. Because of the great increase in pederastry and other exceptional sexual practices in our day, especially in our large metropolitan areas, it seems logical to list these infections of the anal region in the differential diagnosis of venereal disease.

The various diseases affecting the anogenital regions follow under their specific headings.

1. Pyogenic diseases (pus-producing diseases) Impetigo, erysipelas, carbuncles, etc.
2. Dermatomycoses (fungus infections)
3. Animal parasites (crab lice, body lice, scabies, etc.)
4. Filterable viruses (herpes simplex, venereal warts)
5. Aphthosis (ulcerations)
6. Neurodermatitis: pruritus vulvae (itching of the vagina) pruritus ani (itching of the anus) pruritus (itching of the penis and the scrotum)
7. Unclassified: eczema, seborrheic dermatitis, acne vulgaris, edema of the genitals, psoriasis, Lichen planus, Cornu cutaneum
8. Drug eruptions: localized, fixed, anaphylactic reactions
9. Pigmentary changes (hyperpigmentation and depigmentation)
10. Changes in the pubic and genital hair
11. Nutritional deficiencies
12. Genital ulcers (mechanical, thermal, chemical or physical trauma, non-venereal infections,

acute infectious diseases)

13. Diffuse irritative inflammation of the glans, prepuce and vulva
14. Progressive sclerotic atrophic processes of the penis and the vulva
15. Neoplasma (benign and malignant)
16. Lymphatic system diseases. (The nonvenereal bubo, elephantiasis of the lymph glands, and chronic elephantiasis of the vulva)

Such a list demonstrates that almost any disease of the integumentary system may appear in the genital region, and with it occurs all of the confusing distortions attendant upon the regional changes of anatomical and physical pecularities of this area. To the individual experiencing his or her initial herpes of the genitals, venereal warts, crab lice, vulvitis, or any of the genital diseases, however simple, the original fear reaction is just as severe as if the signs were indicative of either syphilis or gonorrhea. Most of the diseases I have listed here respond quickly and efficiently to proper medical care if recognized in time. The physical and mental agonies of the patient can easily be relieved by the doctor's diagnosis and reassurance. Unfortunately, most of these diseases are allowed to flourish out of proportion, and by the time the physician is consulted, the patient has racked himself into a nervous state that impedes the progress of proper cure. In the teaching of sex knowledge, care of the genitals and observation of possible changes are certainly essential. A second step is insistence upon proper medical consultation upon recognition of any change, however slight, in the integrity of the anogenital region of the human body.

As a practicing syphilologist I cannot begin to narrate the accounts of the hundreds of frightened patients whom I have seen who, because of fear associated with sexual activity, have permitted themselves and their genital organs to become maimed when in all probability their problem, before neglect, could have been resolved with prescribed pharmaceutical lotions, powders, compresses, topical antibiotic ointments, antiparasitic medications, steroid creams and the like.

It is in the area of ignorance that many sufferers from the gay deceivers and the minor venereal diseases have endured agony and isolation. There have been many attempts in the past to do away with VD and eliminate its spread. In biblical times, mutilated victims (often persons afflicted with psoriasis or leprosy) were driven from the population and made outcasts. In the Middle Ages this practice continued, and even to the present day we have never been able to shake off a social condemnation of those infected with VD. Our vendetta against syphilis and gonorrhea has extended to the victims of the more ugly "gay deceivers." Any victim of acne vulgaris, psoriasis, or herpes simplex 11 will tell you unbelievable stories of personal suffering because of an unsightly blight upon the skin. The uneducated take one look, shudder and withdraw from any and all forms of physical contact and communication. In the eyes of the observer, the stigma upon the body is inherently "venereal" or "dirty."

It is this attitude of making outcasts of the victims of VD and the mimicking skin ailments which has been largely responsible for the universal lack of cooperation among the masses of people. "A pox upon you," was the Elizabethan cry which is echoed in the infected individual today who passes on the infection "just for spite!"

10

TOMORROW AND TOMORROW AND TOMORROW

In the study of VD, the question will continue to arise . . . *Why not a vaccine?* Before we can answer this question, let us acquaint ourselves with the scientific facts about vaccines, and the general subject of immunization.

Possibly the most widely acclaimed victory of immunology in recent years has been the polio vaccine of the '50s. Until that time, immunizations began and ended with inoculations against smallpox, tetanus, diptheria, typhus, typhoid, and whooping cough. There were a few others—for yellow fever, for example—which were and are employed primarily for use in foreign travel, for the hazards of occupation, and direct contact with the disease. Since the discovery by a team of scientists led by Dr. Jonas Salk, several other important vaccines have been discovered and put to use. The vaccines have been useful largely in the control of virus diseases, including measles, rubella, and mumps.

The unfortunate story of one potentially beneficient vaccine, the vaccine for tuberculosis, is particularly illustrative of the many difficulties that beset the conservative investigator into the prevention of disease. Tragically, the early testing of the vaccine resulted in several deaths in the Scandinavian countries. Thereafter, and particularly in the United States, the vaccine, although basically sound and of infinite potential value, was virtually abandoned for use on a large scale.

Vaccines contain antigenic materials—which means that they stimulate the production of antibodies that react specifically with the antigens. In this respect, the mechanism is similar, in a converse fashion, to that of the allergic reaction involving as it does the interplay of allergens (antigens) and their issue, the reagins (allergic antibodies). One entails an increased capacity to react to the foreign substance (the antigen) and the other a decrease in that capacity.

If the antibody is to be effective in preventing disease, it must match a particular antigenic component of the disease agent which is responsible for the symptoms. There must be enough of the antibody to do this, and it must be present in the body at the correct time.

It is probable that a good vaccine can be developed, for example, against the common cold group of viruses, but one has not yet been discovered because there are just too many different types of responsible viruses for any one vaccine to have been effective. In the "influenza" vaccines, we are dealing primarily with limited types of influenza virus which are subject to mutations that alter them antigenically. A vaccine, therefore, for an outbreak of influenza, is only effective if it matches the genetic type involved in the outbreak. This has been the explanation on the part of doctors and public health officials to administer vaccines that had been developed for one type of flu virus, when another more potent one appeared on the scene.

There are many instances of "cross-immunity," however, where similar antigens may produce antibodies to related diseases, as was the case of the original vaccination where the causative agent of the relatively innocuous cowpox was used to immunize against a much more serious analog, smallpox. On the other hand, vaccines may also consist of weakened or attenuated strains of the disease agent or the elements of those organisms which have been killed by the action of such things as heat or chemicals.

The second most important fact the reader should know relative to vaccine is that the vaccines are most effective when the virus or toxin is present in the circulating blood some time *before* the more serious symptoms of the disease appear. Viruses are the smallest infectious agents, being in effect single molecules but nevertheless much smaller than bacteria. For example, the true viruses—of which diptheria and tetanus are outstanding examples—are often single molecules. As such, both viruses and their toxins are neutralized by antibodies specific for them. The virus becomes noninfectious, the toxin nonpoisonous. The viruses of smallpox and polio and the toxins of diptheria and tetanus do most of their damage after being distributed by the bloodstream. If enough antibody to neutralize the virus or the toxin is *present in the blood before this happens,* the serious symptoms do not develop.

On the other hand, larger cellular agents of disease, including the bacteria, are huge and extremely complex chemically compared with viruses and toxins. Generally speaking a vaccine, or antibodies formed against the mass of antigenic material, hardly ever kills but rather inactivates living, virulent cells.

Incredibly, in the area of VD, the possibility of a vaccine for gonorrhea is being explored. Gonorrhea, by all its characteristics, is as unlikely a candidate as the "common cold" for a good, effective vaccine. The gonococcus has all of the complexity of bacteria and more. It does not enter into the bloodstream until late in the disease; it is the early infectious period of gonorrhea against which we need to establish preventive methods. As with syphilis, there is no natural innate immunity.

Because of the widespread increase in the incidence of gonorrhea, the hope for a discovery of a vaccine has accompanied the very important explorations to develop a blood test for gonorrhea. It has been proven in the VD group in Atlanta, Georgia, that a gonococcus can be grown in culture, and there has been an effort, which has been largely successful, to keep the culture virulent. In this same group there has been an attempt to produce experimental gonorrhea in chimpanzees. Hitherto, no source of gonorrhea has been explored in any other animal than man.

Ironically, the number-one hope for an eventual vaccine for gonorrhea comes from the military. In the army there exist two problem diseases—one is "nice" but often fatal; the other "not nice" but not fatal; the first is cerebrospinal meningitis, the second, gonorrhea. The meningococcus tends to live harmlessly in the throat, and only occasionally breaks through into the blood and then to the lining tissues of the brain called meninges. The meningococcus and the gonococcus are first cousins. What the doctors at Walter Reed Hospital have been trying to develop is a vaccine from the meningococcus while it is living tranquilly in the throat where it is possibly developing a natural immunity. The entire procedure is in an experimental stage, but some of the results look promising.

It is in the area of syphilis, however, that some concentrated work is going on in the development of a vaccine. The technical difficulties are quite different from those of gonorrhea. The spirochete of syphilis cannot be cultured predictably: *Treponema pallidum* grows only in the tissue of man and in a very few, rare species of animal. One of the hopeful features of syphilis is that the disease follows a pattern conducive to the employment of an effective vaccine in that the spirochetes are in the blood very early in the course of the disease, possibly even early enough to prevent the original chancre if the proper immunizing antibody level were high enough at the time of exposure.

Also, certain things happen in syphilis which indicate that there is, at least, a temporary immunity to the disease. For example, in untreated syphilis, or in syphilis that is not treated until several months have elapsed after the first appearance of the symptoms, another exposure does not renew the disease. In the untreated syphilitic, this immunity is obviously because he still is infected. When he is treated later in the disease and cured, there seems to be an immunity for the length of time that the level of circulating antibodies is high enough to insure against infection.

In the prepenicillin days, it was felt that syphilis conferred a lasting immunity, and that the many cases of syphilis recurrence that were seen were "relapses" or "arrested cases." In retrospect, however, these were more likely to have been instances of reinfection occurring in medically cured, or spontaneously burnt-out cases. The conferred immunity, except in cases of congenital syphilis, never seems to have been of such long duration.

To date, we must presume that there exists a temporary immunity to syphilis but its exact nature has not yet been discovered. If we assume there is such a thing as immunity biologically created, then hope for a vaccine is not futile.

The effective vaccine must contain the particular antigen or antigens of the virus, cell, or toxin that gives rise to the antibodies which are protective and which should, therefore, be so treated or diluted so as to be harmless to the individual who receives them. Actually, the ideal vaccine would contain nothing else, but no vaccine has achieved such purity. There is always an imminent danger to the recipient, even in such established vaccines as the smallpox vaccine, which is taken for granted by most people: The scar produced by the cowpox virus, discovered by Edward Jenner, seems for the most part to be a small price to pay for the avoidance of smallpox, but there are, even at this date, some deaths reported resulting from the vaccine. If a vaccine were developed for syphilis it would certainly have to be mild, hopefully harmless, characteristically distinct from syphilis and incapable of turning into syphilis. Otherwise the vaccine would be worthless, in addition to being sufficiently dangerous to scare people away from its use.

In 1968, the Mexican Institute of Health and Tropical Diseases discovered that the pinta spirochete is occasionally infectious for chimpanzees. Pinta is not a serious disease, but its bleached lesions are regarded as disfiguring, especially by dark-complexioned people. However, if the vaccine could be developed from the pinta spirochete as effective against syphilis, the contracting of an abortive case of pinta would be regarded by most people as a satisfactory price to pay. The number-one obstacle in the research on this vaccine is that pinta is a slow-developing disease—slower even possibly than syphilis, so that the probability of using it to immunize against syphilis seems rather remote at this stage. Another spirochete being investigated as a possible vaccine is one found in the African monkey which has been shown closely to resemble the spirochete of yaws. This experiment is also in the primitive stages as very little is known about the behavior of the spirochete in animals other than monkeys.

In addition to the possible discovery of vaccines to combat the problem of VD, there have been some technological studies, notably, the use of the gamma-ray irradiation that destroys the virulence of the spirochetes, but does not, so far, stop their movement. Rabbits innoculated with such irradiated treponemas developed both reagin-type and immobolizing antibodies without showing symptoms. When virulent spirochetes were later injected into the skin these animals appeared to be immune. However, this test has not yet been used on man.

In Nevada, where prostitution is legal, one pharmaceutical company is conducting a study under carefully controlled conditions with state and federal government acknowledgment, of a drug which at this stage shows high promise as a VD preventative. The drug is an oily liquid substance known as Progonasyl. A few drops of Progonasyl (an organic iodine previously used to treat vaginal inflammation, nose and ear infections, and as a presurgical preparation of membranes), is inserted into the vagina. Following a brief rest period—five to ten minutes—protection can be expected for the subsequent twenty-four hours.

During this study conducted with the all-volunteer cooperation of the prostitutes in twenty of about forty legal brothels in Nevada, only two girls contracted gonorrhea, and this was very likely due to the fact that they missed the required daily dosage. Nevada State Health Officer Dr. John H. Carr found that many of the prostitutes involved refuse to have intercourse without the daily dosage. "From the data we've collected this far we feel we can say the drug is an effective preventative. There have been no dangerous side effects, although about ten percent of the girls have withdrawn from the program because Progonasyl created some irritations."

Amerex Laboratories, developers of Progonasyl, point out that the drug is still in the investigative stage. Nevertheless it is encouraging that both government agencies and private industry are cognizant of the fact that something must be done to halt, obliterate, and in the future prevent the ever increasing menace of VD.

Interestingly enough, the discovery by Dr. Sabin of the possible link between the herpetic ulcer and cancer may be cause for future advancement, because it links VD to a disease that is not only a terrible plague for mankind, but a disease to which much medical research and unlimited financial funds have been allotted for prevention, cure, and public enlightenment.

Actually, VD suffers from financial impoverishment both from government agencies and private endowment. There is great need for educational propaganda informing the public how to recognize VD as a medical problem and not a moral problem; and an overall need for a reeducation of the sexual habits of the oncoming generation to know everything possible about VD. And, obviously, there is a need for the financing of research to discover both a simpler means of diagnosis for gonorrhea—either blood test, skin test, or bacterial slide—and a vaccine both for syphilis and gonorrhea. Meanwhile, we have to cope with the material we have at our disposal and make the most intelligent use of the tools that are available.

Certainly if a VD vaccine were discovered, there would be a major problem of inducing the public to submit voluntarily to such a vaccination—even if it were proven to be absolutely harmless. A privately conducted survey amongst patients and acquaintances proved most interesting. There was a small group of very liberated modern-thinking parents who jumped enthusiastically at the suggestion and said they would immediately have their children—and themselves—vaccinated if such a vaccine existed; there was a second group that had experienced some difficulties with sundry "influenza" vaccines that had proven either ineffective or more sickening than the actual "flu"—at least in their opinions; a third group was skeptical of anything regarding VD vaccines as a result of the ineffectiveness of penicillin in eradicating the diseases; and a fourth group, which I am afraid we shall, like the poor, have with us always, that in some mystical manner believe that VD will never touch them—Tom Jones, Mary Smith, yes—but me, Bill Brown, *never!* Whether their sublime faith is based upon ignorance or ancient inbred religious beliefs that VD is a punishment for sexual sin, no one can determine.

Among parents with whom I discussed the problem, most of the attitudes revolved upon their experience with "the pill," with drugs, and with their children. Most admitted being confronted with a new generation that seemed determined to pursue its own way, based upon the logical reasoning that the ways of their forebears had not produced a way of life that intrigued them. Parents who refused to give their daughters the required parental consent for use of the pill awoke to discover that daughter had either obtained a prescription without their consent or become involved in the problems of abortion, adoption, or shot-gun marriage followed by early divorce. In the final analysis, parents had to accept the fact that sex, like drugs, had "reared its ugly head," and the manifestation in a sexually permissive society presented problems with which they had not been trained to cope.

Until VD prevention becomes reality, most doctors continue to suggest to patients that they rely upon simple commonsense measures to aid them in warding off infection. Such measures should be considered mandatory if one's sexual partner is a stranger or a casual, hastily encountered acquaintance. In such encounters, the old-fashioned condom should be used, and used in its original context, *to prevent venereal disease.* If the sex partner is a woman and is on the pill, the man should be alerted to use the condom for this original intent. If the man is reluctant then the woman should insist upon it. A person, male or female, should cleanse themselves thoroughly, externally and internally, following a random sexual encounter. Soap and water may not be the positive to a great number of germs, but they do wash away quite a few. A woman should shower and scrub her pubic area with soap and water. This procedure also will help eliminate such bothersome venereal problems as crab lice. And she should douche.

The reader may complain that the romance and magic of sex are destroyed by having to use such crude, practical methods of prevention of VD. But the hard-core facts offset fantasy. As a friend commented, "reality aches." There is nothing romantic about the gift a venereally infected human being passes on to another. And, there is less and less romance and glamour attached to the chain of events of exposure which follow. The protective routine prescribed here is the one in which intelligent prostitutes engage after coupling with a customer. Since the prostitute has no emotional involvement but a livelihood at stake, the routine is a sensible and practical one which has sustained her in her profession. Until a better resolution comes along, perhaps, it is the reasonable formula to follow.

Today, the major thrust of the war against VD, is in the combat hands of the public-health authorities. Some of the work done is commendable, such as the fact that anyone can be treated in a public-health VD clinic *without charge.* The basic flaw with the public-health system is that it is committed to a follow-up policy that seems logical on paper, but is not too workable in actual practice.

Public-health officials believe that treating an infected person is not enough; they are cognizant of the fact that they must track down the source of the patient's infection and extend treatment to that person also. Accordingly, everyone treated at a public-health facility is asked to cooperate by providing the names of his or her recent sexual contacts. Similarly, every doctor is required by law to report all cases of VD to the public-health department and the patients involved are expected to cooperate so that the contacts can be identified, sought out and treated. On paper it looks very orderly and proper, but it depends entirely on the vagaries of human beings and their often stunted sense of public responsibility.

So what?

It is quite possible that we could solve the matter of the control of syphilis *if we wanted to.* This is a control without new technique, control based upon the knowledge we have on hand. The specific requirements are:

> 1) The American Medical Association must recognize the need for more comprehensive study for medical students on the subject of syphilis so that knowledge of the medical, social, and public-health aspects of VD may be taught by actual clinical contact with patients under the direction of qualified teachers. As the watchdog of medical

education in the United States, the AMA should ascertain the standards of teaching programs in dermatology and syphilology in all medical schools, making sure that previously recognized deficient teaching programs are rectified and kept abreast of scientific and sociological advances.

2) With better training of practicing doctors, a full-fledged educational program for continued study be made available with symposia for the exclusive study of venereal diseases and syphilology.

3) More and better clinics with improved facilities for diagnosis and treatment, including properly trained VD personnel.

4) Development of a comprehensive and dynamic education program for professional workers and general public. This program should range from physicians to schoolchildren.

5) Intensification and extension of current interview-investigation services to cover all infectious syphilis cases.

6) Continuation of research in syphilis immunology, therapy, and laboratory procedure and greater expansion of research in adolescent and young adult sexual behavior.

7) Unstinted cooperation of support by federal, state, and local governments of efforts made by the private practitioner, and equal cooperation of the private physician with the agencies established to help control and eradicate syphilis.

8) Honest concern about the problem ranging from the highest officials to the simplest member of society with no emphasis on shame or punishment.

In syphilis we must face the fact that the tools, knowledge, epidemiologic methodology, and technical know-how to detect, cure, and prevent syphilis cases are now available. As a private practicing physician I must call myself and my fellow doctors to task in relation to the control of syphilis. One of the most important elements in the syphilis control program in the United States is the participation of private physicians who still treat more syphilitic patients in their offices than are treated in public clinics. Unfortunately, private physicians *do not report all their cases to the health department.* In 1968, a national survey carried out by the American Social Health Association indicated that private physicians reported only 19 percent of their infectious syphilitic patients to the health department.

Today the Venereal Disease Branch of the Public Health Department is attempting to improve the participation of private physicians in syphilis control. Representatives of the health department visit doctors to stimulate case reporting and to encourage physicians to request health-department assistance in bringing source and spread contacts to medical attention. When a patient with a reactive serologic test is reported by a laboratory, the physician is often visited to ensure that the case receives a medical disposition and that a case report is submitted if indicated. New practicing physicians are also requested to cooperate with the control program.

In fairness to the private physician, the patient, and the investigating public health official, there are certain truths which should be surfaced. The practicing private physician is inculcated from the beginning with the "sacredness" of the relationship that has existed between doctor and patient since the days of Hippocrates. The violation of a patient's confidence does, indeed, offend almost every dedicated doctor I have ever known. On the other hand, there is not a "dedicated" syphilologist either, with whom I have studied and worked, who has not been fully cognizant that the basic control of VD lies in the knowledge of the source of original contact and the knowledge of contacts made following infection. However, the situation is so tenuous that once the disease is diagnosed by the doctor, the intimate and essential doctor-patient relationship is very often shattered. In many cases the patient disappears and seeks help elsewhere, convinced that his doctor is "out to get him."

The number of instances when the original diagnosis of VD by a private practicing physician has resulted in an unpaid bill and a loss of the patient, have been the source of much consternation among syphilologists. In many cases, the doctor has resolved that his knowledge of the disease is such that he can forestall the eventual agonies in his patient, and has rationalized that one cure is worth the price of secrecy; he does not report the case to the health authorities because he had believed that to do so will not only cause the patient to leave, but that the health authorities would not have been any more successful than he in ferreting out his patient's contacts.

The other factor involved is the established physician's distrust and dislike of government in the field of medicine. Like lawyers, teachers, and blacksmiths, in the early days of medicine in America, the doctor was often paid in barters of food, land, and occasional thanks. Without government aid, he barged ahead and organized to eradicate the quacks, to establish standards for medical institutions to protect the health of the masses of people. That there was no original cooperation between the doctor and government as government pursued a policy of laissez faire, is one of the many tragedies of medicine in our society, to the detriment of public health; and government interference came with such catastrophic speed that doctors became most adamant in their resentment of any government intervention and fearful that it would extend into their practice and the privacy of their doctor-patient relationships. The modern doctor is straddling a difficult issue to resolve, and VD control is one of the best diseases to illustrate the predicament of all concerned.

Unquestionably, there are many officious and, very often,

medically ignorant public-health officials who, because they represent the law, invade the rights of the private practicing doctor and the rights of his patient. Most of my colleagues and I have experienced such encounters. In instances of intelligent understanding and cooperation, most of the problems involved can be resolved, but the few that are handled badly create more impact than those well handled.

There are many reasons for lack of communication between public-health officials, doctors in private practice and patients. One of the most important is the scarcity of both doctors and public-health officials and, especially, the scarcity of those who are trained in the psychological aspects of the problems involved. All people concerned are overworked, weary of coping with what appears to be an insurmountable problem. Tired nerves give way, logic and mutual understanding are lost, communication ceases, and hostilities emerge. The result is an ever increasing breach between the very important public-health officials and the private practicing doctor and his patients who seek him out for the very fact of his cognomen—*private.*

Obviously syphilis surveillance involves an extensive serologic testing program among such diverse groups as premarital applicants, pregnant females, blood donors, hospital admissions, men and women examined for or discharged from the military service, alleged contacts to known infectious cases, employment and pre-employment examinations, and persons undergoing examinations in physicians' offices. Except in seronegative primary syphilis, a reactive test nearly always precedes a diagnosis of syphilis. In order to maximize the contribution of the serologic screening network to syphilis control in the United States, a law was passed in 1962 requiring every laboratory performing serologic tests for syphilis to notify the health department of each reactive specimen tested giving the name of the patient and the attending physician.

Of the 38,000,000 blood specimens examined annually in the United States, about 1,100,000 are reactive for syphilis. Of the total number reactive 800,000 (73%) are reported to health departments. Follow-up of these reactors results in approximately 10,000 case reports of infectious syphilis and 62,000 reports of syphilis in other stages. Infectious-syphilis patients are interviewed, and when possible their sex contacts are brought to medical examination and treatment. Theoretically, the source and spread of the disease could be under control; it is the "when possible" clause which alters the conditions of the action from active to passive.

But the case for syphilis control today—and tomorrow—is not beyond hope even if science does not advance one stage further than it has today. It is contained within the realm of individual intelligence and available knowledge and access to medical facilities.

The case for control of gonorrhea is much less heartening. Gonorrhea is now pandemic and found in all walks of life—especially among the young—a million and a half new cases per year is a conservative estimate in the United States alone. It ranks first among reportable communicable diseases. The pandemic is clearly out of hand and the medical problems entailed in bringing it under control are vast. As we know, detection is much more difficult than is generally supposed. Most people are loathe to seek treatment. Physicians have a traditionally "low index" of suspicion in looking for an asymptomatic infection. And, the gonococcus is finding new hiding places, such as the pharynx and the anal canal, neither of which is either examined or cultured routinely.

Even worse, the development of strains with high resistance to penicillin and to alternative antibiotics has nightmare implications. In the past three decades the required dose of penicillin for acute uncomplicated gonorrhea has increased from 75,000 units to 4.8 million units—64 times as much. And, today, the required dose is often double that of just a few years ago. The prospect of any decrease in the incidence of gonorrhea seems dismal indeed. A vaccine seems many years off, if it is possible at all. An encouraging tool for doctors to work with today is the development of media to enable all practitioners to diagnose gonorrhea readily by culture. However, if a person is *known* to have been exposed to gonorrhea, he should be treated regardless of physical findings, and without cultural proof of infection, for the culture occasionally does miss the infection. Early treatment also will hopefully eliminate further spread between the time of culture and culture confirmation. Treatment, therefore, is more on an epidemiological than on a soundly scientific medical basis.

Frequently, we hear of a woman who has gone to her doctor because she discovered her boyfriend has been treated for gonorrhea. After a negative physical and stained smear, the girl is told there is no infection present. Actually, such a case should be cultured and preferably treated for gonorrhea, because the Gram stain on the female frequently only misleads the physician.

A major aspect of control is public education. Too much emphasis cannot be placed upon the importance of gonorrhea, its symptoms and its *lack* of them! The patient is urged to seek treatment early. It is true that doctors report only one out of eight or ten cases of gonorrhea treated. This is understandable, since once reported, it is just a statistic. No contact investigation is done as a rule, and the patient's contacts are not brought in for treatment. In essence, the doctor is turning in some private patient's name as having had a disease that has a social stigma attached. Consequently, reporting gonorrhea by case seems unimportant in defining the scope of the overall problem.

Since there exists no reliable serologic screening test for gonorrhea, there seems to be little hope that gonorrhea will be controlled with the present available methods.

Except for the work at a few medical schools, clinics, and laboratories, very little research on either syphilis or gonorrhea is being done. We have pointed out the efforts—which are minute in comparison to the vast research done in other diseases. The picture is most unfortunate and with the widespread incidence of VD today there is a great need for an endowment of vast proportions. In addition to funds for vaccine and serologic tests, there is additional need for educational funds. For the time being this need exceeds the research need, for we desperately require some immediate solution. If treated properly, syphilis and gonorrhea, if caught in time, can be cured. Since this condition exists, why have these diseases gotten out of control? Largely, through ignorance and negligence.

We need a program of venereal-disease education aimed at the general public. All forms of mass media should be involved, including radio, TV (the Dick Cavett Emmy award-winning show was an example of how the subject can be treated in a form of entertainment that will attract the age group most involved), films, newspapers, magazines, billboards, and car cards. Literature with information of available treatment centers should be posted in areas of contact, such as the lavatories of bars and massage parlors, and in public meeting places. Programmed instruction books for teachers and pupils in elementary and high schools should be distributed, read, and openly discussed as to content and meaning. The main purpose of this program should be to teach the student to recognize the signs and symptoms to seek medical attention immediately if in doubt.

Too much emphasis cannot be placed upon the fact that the beauty and romance of sex is over, when the malady lingers on!

In the final analysis, our hope for tomorrow is based upon a large allocation of money for public education, medical research for a vaccine for syphilis, a serologic test for gonorrhea and, possibly, a vaccine. In addition to these needs, we need the cooperation of the individual with private physicians and established VD health centers. Our shame is not venereal disease per se, but our ignorant attacks on the disease that perpetuates its existence.

11

QUESTIONS AND ANSWERS

1. What is VD?

The letters VD stand for venereal disease which is contracted through sexual contact with the vagina, the penis, the anus, and the mouth. Syphilis and gonorrhea are the most prevalent and most serious of the venereal diseases although there are others less well known.

2. How is VD contracted?

VD, specifically syphilis and gonorrhea, is peculiar to humans and is contracted by men and women in sexual encounters with other infected men or women. Any other source of contagion is very rare, and is usually socially devised myth for face-saving purposes only.

3. Why are syphilis and gonorrhea called "social diseases?"

Syphilis and gonorrhea have a sociological impact and meaning as well as a medical one. For example, VD and prostitution have been bedfellows since the beginning of time. Even today, prostitution, both male and female, is the number-one source of VD infection.

4. What is the solution to the epidemic aspects of VD?
More explicit sex education. Removal of the mid-Victorian "shame" aspect of the diseases. Open and frank sex discussions regarding the diseases. Releasing of sources of contacts to control the rapid spread of VD.

5. Who gets VD?
No one is invulnerable. The more sexually promiscuous are more prone to get VD and also to pass the diseases on to unsuspecting partners. Young people and middle aged. Heterosexuals and homosexuals. Drug addicts. People who are careless and ignorant. People all over the world, although the incidence is higher in cities than in rural areas and higher in some countries than in others.

6. Do animals have syphilis?
No. The incidences reported of syphilis among sheep and llamas are of human origin and the disease is not transmitted from an infected animal to another animal.

7. Is penicillin a cure for VD?
Penicillin is a specific for VD when properly administered in sufficiently large doses. It can be a cure, providing the patient follows through with the prescribed medical program.

8. With penicillin a specific, why is there a current VD epidemic?
Because no system of control of VD exists. Control requires a vaccine for syphilis and gonorrhea and a serologic test for gonorrhea, neither of which have yet been discovered.

9. Are current vital statistics factual?
No, the increase in VD is undoubtedly much greater than the available statistics.

10. Where did syphilis originate?

The origin of syphilis is as controversial today as it was in the first epidemic occurrences of the disease. Some scholars support the theory that the disease was brought by Columbus and his sailors when they returned to the continent of Europe following the first expedition to the new world; others, that the disease existed since beginning of the history of man.

11. What is the cause of syphilis?

The organism of syphilis, the spirochete, *Treponema pallidum,* is a spirillum requiring moisture and tissue for survival. It is peculiar to human beings and is transferred by means of sexual contact.

12. How is syphilis recognized?

In the first stage, by a hard chancre appearing on the penis, the vulva, the anus, or the mouth; in the second stage, by a rash that can appear anywhere on the body and lasts but a few days, usually accompanied by fever and a severe headache; in the third stage, by physical and personality changes such as locomotor ataxia, cardiovascular disturbances, severe headaches, blindness, convulsive rages; and in the final stage, by paresis and death.

13. What should a person suspecting syphilis do?

First and foremost, if a person suspects the presence of syphilis, all sexual contacts should be avoided until a comprehensive medical examination is performed. If the prognosis is positive, all recent sexual contacts up to a period of six months should be notified and urged to seek an examination. Consult a doctor immediately. In the first two stages, a syphilologist (dermatologist), in the later stages, a urologist, an internist, or neurologist depending upon the area of suspicion. In any event a doctor should be consulted because, while the therapy with penicillin is relatively simple, the diagnosis is very complicated. If one cannot afford a private physician for consultation, a Public Health VD clinic or a special VD clinic supported by private funds are available.

14. Is syphilis inherited?
No. Congenital syphilis is the passing of the infection from the syphilitic mother to the fetus in the womb, and the infant is born with syphilis.

15. If one contracted syphilis as a youth, was treated with penicillin, and is unsure whether the cure was effective or not, what should be done?
Any person having had syphilis should have periodic examinations and serologic blood tests. One never develops an immunity to syphilis unless one is a congenital syphilitic. Any radical personality changes and symptomatic physical ailments should be checked and the doctor notified of the past history of syphilis. The changes, or the appearance of neurosyphilis, occur anywhere from ten to thirty years after the original infection. The only completely satisfactory diagnosis of neurosyphilis is an examination of the spinal fluid.

16. What is the cause of gonorrhea?
Gonorrhea is caused by the gonococcus, a member of the common class of parasitic bacteria that has cohabited with man since the beginning of time. It is transmitted by sexual contact.

17. What are the symptoms?
The symptoms can be complicated—especially in women, and homosexuals with anal or pharyngeal gonorrhea. Within twenty-four or forty-eight hours to ten or fifteen days in the male the symptoms can occur, namely discharge of pus, painful urination from the penis and urinary tract. Medical diagnosis is made by examining the discharge under a microscope where the appearance of the typically paired gonococci

inside the pus-cells identify the disease. In the more difficult and unusual manifestations, diagnosis is often difficult and sometimes painful and not always effective.

18. If one suspects gonorrhea, what should one do?
Seek medical help immediately. Do not try home remedies or well-meaning friend's suggestions. A woman should seek out a gynecologist, a man a urologist. If the pus should first appear in the eyes a dermatologist-syphilologist or an opthalomologist. Avoid all sexual contacts, and notify any recent sex partners to see a doctor as well.

19. Do animals have gonorrhea?
No. The disease is peculiar to human beings. It can be transmitted through sexual contact and to the infant from the mother at birth. There is no immunity and the disease can be contracted so long as one continues to have sexual contacts which carry the disease.

20. What is the treatment for gonorrhea?
A number of antibiotics can be used successfully. Despite the increase of antibiotic resistant organisms, it is still possible to cure gonorrhea with sufficiently high levels of penicillin.

21. What are the dangers of gonorrhea when untreated?
Sterility. In women if the Fallopian tubes have become seriously infected they have to be removed. Endocarditis, meningitis, arthritis, and septic joints are also serious complications.

22. Is the disease more peculiar to one sex? One race?
Gonorrhea is more difficult to diagnose in women because of the lack of a serological test, and a woman can have the disease for a long time before becoming aware of her infection. One peculiarity is that women using oral contraceptives

are one-half times more likely to get gonorrhea from a single exposure to an infected partner than a woman who does not use them. The reason given is that the pill must alter the pH of the vagina and predispose the patient to infection.

The suggestion that black races get a more severe or more infectious case of gonorrhea is purely a myth. Actually the reason for this speculation is based upon bias. Poverty and ignorance of sex hygiene and facts relative to gonorrhea that cause delay in seeking medical help, make the infection more deeply rooted when medical help is sought, and penicillin less effective.

23. What is required to control gonorrhea?
A better serological test, a safer and more effective antibiotic, a vaccine and possibly a disinfectant vaginal cream. The finding of a susceptible animal in the chimpanzee for experimentation would alter the entire future in the cure and control of gonorrhea.

24. What are the dangers of VD in pregnancy?
In syphilis, the infant is protected during the early months in the fetal form from acquiring syphilis from the mother. After the fifth month the danger to the mother and the unborn infant occurs resulting in miscarriage, premature birth and if unattended a congenitally syphilitic offspring.

In gonorrhea the danger to the infant is at birth where the eyes are most vulnerable.

25. What treatments should the pregnant mother and infant receive?
Dosages of penicillin before and at birth when the serologic tests are positive. The congenitally syphilitic baby properly treated and observed from birth to adolescence can often avoid the disastrous pitfalls of the disease.

26. What should a pregnant girl do?

Obviously have her pregnancy diagnosed as soon as possible and if VD is present follow her obstetrician's care. Pre-natal and post-natal check-ups are stressed for both mother and infant. If the gravid woman cannot afford private medical care she should as soon as she suspects pregnancy apply for free medical assistance at the clinics designated for such care.

27. Why should one consult a doctor?

Because the presence of any lesion or discharge—especially in the sex organs—should be diagnosed professionally because the possibility of VD is always present. Until a proper diagnosis is given, one can worry needlessly. If the diagnosis is positive, obviously medical care and attention must be administered.

INDEX